P9-EFJ-379

Cultural Diversity in Health and Illness

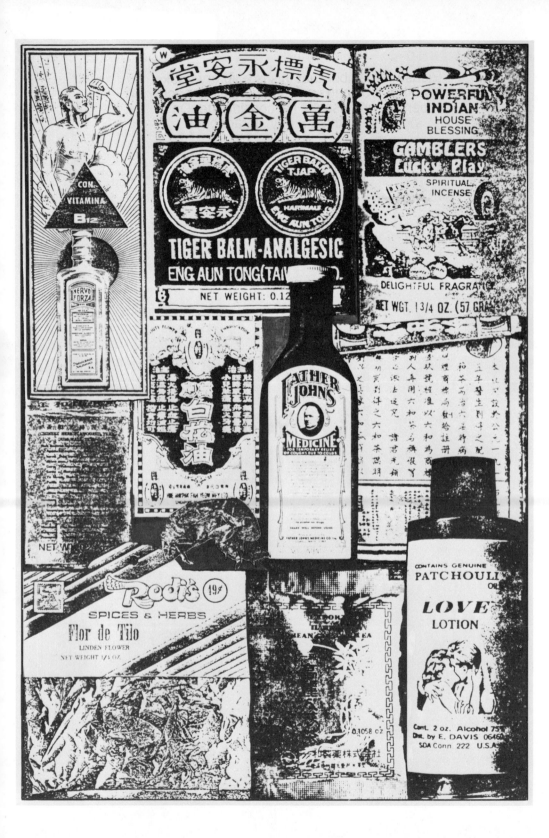

Cultural Diversity in Health and Illness

Rachel E. Spector, R.N., M.S.

Assistant Professor Boston College School of Nursing
Chestnut Hill, Massachusetts

With contributions by

Manuel Spector, M.S.W., M.S. Hyg., Ph.D.
Special Consultant
Immigration and Naturalization Service
Formerly
Assistant Professor of Social Work
Salem State College
Salem, Massachusetts

Irving Kenneth Zola, Ph.D.
Professor, Sociology
Brandeis University
Waltham, Massachusetts

ĀCC   Appleton-Century-Crofts/New York

80 81 82 83 / 10 9 8 7 6 5 4 3 2

Prentice-Hall International, Inc., London
Prentice-Hall of Australia, Pty. Ltd., Sydney
Prentice-Hall of India Private Limited, New Delhi
Prentice-Hall of Japan, Inc., Tokyo
Prentice-Hall of Southeast Asia (Pte.) Ltd., Singapore
Whitehall Books Ltd., Wellington, New Zealand

Library of Congress Cataloging in Publication Data

Spector, Rachel E., 1940-
    Cultural diversity in health and illness.

    Bibliography: p.
    Includes index.
    1.   Social medicine.   2.   Medical anthropology.
3.   Health attitudes.   4.   Medical personnel and
patient.   5.   Medical care—United States.
6.   Minorities—Health and hygiene—United States.
I.   Title.
RA418.S75   362.2'04'2   79-1470
ISBN 0-8385-1394-8

The quotation on page 4 is from René Dubos, *Mirage of Health*, copyright © 1959 by
René Dubos, with the permission of Harper & Row, Publishers, Inc.

Text design: Karin Batten
Cover design: Susan F. Rich

PRINTED IN THE UNITED STATES OF AMERICA

Contents

Preface

The purpose of this book is to sensitize the reader to the profound dimensions and complexities involved in caring for people from diverse cultural backgrounds. I wish to share with the reader my experiences and thoughts concerning the introduction of cultural concepts into the education of health-care professionals. This book represents one answer to the questions: "How does one effectively expose a student to cultural diversity?" and "How does one examine health-care issues and perceptions from a broad social viewpoint?" As I have done in the classroom, I will attempt to bring the reader into a direct interface between the American health-care system and the consumer of health care.

Today's health-care provider, for the most part, is typically a white person of middle-class background. The consumer presented here is the ethnic person of color—including the Black, the Asian, the Hispanic and the Native American (Indian). There is a twofold purpose for the selection of this population: they are the *least* represented within the health-care delivery system and they tend to experience the greatest difficulty in interacting with health-care providers.

I am neither a sociologist nor an anthropologist, but as a nurse and educator I am committed to finding a way to integrate the concepts of these disciplines into patient care. This book is an attempt to demonstrate several resources and techniques that have proved effective in presenting cultural content to future and present providers of health-care services. To this end, an annotated bibliography has been provided throughout to encourage further exploration into the appropriate literature. Further, the question: "Is health care a right?" is deeply explored and argued. Finally, the text demonstrates suggested ways that one can adapt health-care delivery to meet the needs of the consumer.

Those who provide health care in the remainder of the 1970s and into the 1980s are faced with a changing system of delivery. To ensure safe and effective service to the consumer, it has become the mandate of these times to provide the student and health-care professional with both a technical and cultural educational background. Just as the society is changing, the milieu in which one practices health care is changing. No longer is the consumer willing to "receive" care; rather, the client desires the opportunity to participate in his or her care-related decisions. No longer can the provider dictate a regimen; efforts must be made to collaborate with the consumer in determining a treatment plan. Unless the provider has a sound understanding of the consumer's personal values and perceptions regarding health and illness, he or she is unable to meet the consumer's needs satisfactorily.

The essential argument of this book is that the provider of health care (nurse, physician, social worker, etc.) has been socialized into a distinct provider culture. This provider culture instills in its members its own norms regarding health and illness. When a member of this culture interacts with a person from a culture with differing norms, there is often a conflict in their beliefs. For this reason, I will explore issues of health and illness in four dimensions:

1. Provider self-awareness;
2. Consumer-oriented issues surrounding delivery and acceptance of health care;
3. Broad issues such as poverty (a barrier) and health care as a right (a bridge);
4. Examples of traditional health beliefs and practices among selected populations.

There is much to be learned. Books and articles have begun to appear which address these problems and issues. It is not easy to alter attitudes and beliefs or stereotypes and prejudices. Some social psychologists state that it is almost impossible to lose all of one's prejudices. Yet alterations can be made. I believe the health-care provider must develop a sensitivity to his or her own fundamental values regarding health and illness. With acceptance of one's own values comes the framework and courage to accept the existence of differing values. This process of realization and acceptance can enable the health-care provider to be instrumental in meeting the needs of the consumer in a collaborative, safe, and professional manner.

Acknowledgments

There are several people I wish to thank for their guidance and professional support: Elsie Basque, Joe Colorado, Dean Mary Dineen, Noreen Dresser, Terrie Fermino, Louise-Orlando Isaza, Patricia McArdle, and Irving Zola. I am also grateful to students who have taken the course upon which this text is based; they have generously contributed their thoughts, feelings, and experiences in hopes that the material would come alive for readers. I should like to mention a few of these students by name: Louise Buchanan, Miriam Cook, Vicki Kello, Diane Neely, Valerie Lewis, and Wayne Kelly who provided me with much of the anecdotal material in Chapter 10.

Many thanks also to those friends who tolerated me during the long summer of 1977; to Rosetta Gerry Johnson, former student, current colleague, and friend, who assisted with the initial draft of this text; and to the typists, Michele Wojciechowski and Delores Malloy—as if by magic they always had everything ready on time.

I especially thank Leslie Boyer, my editor. If it were not for her encouragement and understanding, this book would not be a reality. Emily Sisley also deserves special mention for her sensitive and expert editing of the manuscript.

Most of all, I want to acknowledge
the support of my husband and family
and dedicate this volume
To Manny, Sam, Becky
and my parents

Introduction

The historic events of the 1960s have made our society aware of gaps that divide the multitudes of people comprising the American population. In the aftermath of the events that shook the country—e.g., political assassinations, student uprisings, the civil-rights movement, and riots in Watts, Detroit, and Washington, D.C.—the focus on inequality has also entered the arena of health and health-care delivery. Just as other populations now articulate their needs, health-care consumers demand to participate in and understand their care.

Essentially, we have had to find a way of caring for the client that matches the client's perception of the health problem and treatment of that problem. In many situations, this is not difficult; in other situations, it seems impossible. However, with the passage of time, a pattern emerges: for the health-care provider, the client needs most difficult to meet are those of people who are the most "different" from the nurse. These people tend to be ethnic people of color—blacks, Asians, Hispanics, and native American Indians.

In the countless situations in which there is conflict between the provider's and client's belief systems, the provider is typically unable to understand the conflict and, hence, usually finds ways of minimizing it. Ordinarily, the provider knows too little about the way a client views himself, what the client believes about a given situation, and what the client's beliefs are regarding health and illness. For the provider, all that is important is knowing the "hows" and scientific "whys." In the past, little was known of the impact that this kind of attitude had on the recipient of health care. Today we realize that this attitude has had a negative impact on the consumer; thus, the issue is crucial.

The providers are usually aware of—but generally have difficulty relating to—the personal and social problems of these people: such as unemployment, underemployment, welfare, the presence of illegitimate children, and drug and alcohol abuse, to mention only a few. Even though problems of this sort may well account in part for a client's inability to cope with or to follow any kind of medical regimen, little or nothing has been taught professionals in reference to the underlying components of these situations and how they affected the patient or how the patient related to them.

This book will help the reader to take a good look at the macro issues within the context of health and health-care delivery. One must ask: How does the client view life? What are his beliefs, values, and norms? What is his cultural background and how does it influence his behavior? How do such factors affect the *meanings* of "health" and "illness"? What does it all mean in terms of survival? (How does one person's socialization differ from that of another?)

When one completes an educational program and dons the attire of the profession—for example, the traditional white dress and cap of the nurse—little thought is given to one's infallibility. One is now sanctioned by society to enter into the world and deliver the practiced and learned skills. One does not choose to answer to the client who fails to follow the treatment regimen of a physician and/or nurse, who does not keep appointments, or who does not seek early health care. Once licensed, the provider feels secure in the scientific knowledge that took so long to master: Does he or she not "know it all?" The person who fails to comply with treatment, does not attend a clinic appointment, or delays in seeking health care is of little concern. Surely it is not the provider's fault that these situations continue to occur and recur. Surely the fault must lie with the consumer. We continue to rationalize, to look for scapegoats, and most often wind up by labeling the client as "lazy" or "stupid." In the narrowly defined world of the health-care provider, there is only room for blaming the client—who, in this instance, is the *victim*.

According to health-care providers, there are no alternative forms of healing; there are no other healers. The American health-care provider has been socialized to believe that modern medicine as taught and practiced in Western civilization is the answer to *all* of humankind's needs. Has not modern medicine transcended all other forms of healing in technological skills and scientific understanding? With these extraordinary skills and this scientific sophistication, to cite an example, the dead can be brought back to life. When a heart or kidney fails, it can be replaced—either by a machine or by a transplanted organ. Of course, in the eyes of some consumers, Western medicine does not reign omnipotent, and the provider—with social, political, and humanistic concern—observes this phenomenon in diverse ways. For there are countless people who do not follow prescribed regimens; who fail to maintain attendance at a clinic, that is, who "elope" (the term used when a person fails to return to a clinic where he is undergoing treatment); or who spurn medical services or seek them as a last resort, and then leave the health system as quickly as possible. WHY?

The answers are deep and complex. The situations are not new; the answers do not present themselves with ease. In fact, the range of possible explanations is infinite. Sometimes people fail to seek care or to take medication because they cannot afford to purchase the services or the medicine. The question one might then ask is: Why don't health-care seekers accept the care or medicine when it is given to them? I suggest that a deeper level is operative; perhaps the consumer believes that the care and medicine that are offered cannot help him. Perhaps the consumer believes that the offered care makes him sicker or that a given regimen is incompatible with his illness. Until recently in the preparation to practice nursing, medicine, or any other health-care profession, a student was not taught that a client may believe that the regimen or the medication that health care provides is incompatible with his illness. Much of this "incompatibility" is rooted in the almost diametrically opposed views the client and provider may have in perceiving a given health problem. It stands to reason that, if a problem is not perceived in an agreed-upon way, the prescribed treatments may well not be complied with. One source of such perceptual incompatibility lies within one's culturally and ethnically determined perception of the health condition as a given problem.

Those who deliver health care may ask the following questions: "Why, with today's knowledge and communication, doesn't everybody know about and believe in germs and viruses?" "Doesn't everybody know about epidemiology?" "Who has never heard of depression and schizophrenia?" "Is there anyone who doesn't believe in penicillin and thorazine?" "Shouldn't everybody believe in and practice prevention and public health?" "What is there to believe in if not the medical model of disease?"

I believe that there is a fundamental difference between the health beliefs of health care providers and the consumers. Indeed, there are numerous beliefs that underlie our practices in both health and illness. Many (if not all) of these beliefs are set in motion and de-

termined by our socio-cultural-ethnic backgrounds. In the forth-
coming pages I intend to develop the following arguments:

1. That each person enters the health professions with
   culturebound definitions of health and illness;
2. That we bring with us distinct practices for the
   prevention and treatment of illness;
3. That our ideas change as we are socialized into the
   "health-care provider culture";
4. That a schism of various degrees develops between
   the provider of health services and the recipient of
   these services; and,
5. That if the provider becomes more sensitive to the
   issues surrounding health care and the traditional
   health beliefs of the consumer, he or she will be
   enabled to provide far more comprehensive health
   care.

I am able to validate this theory with analyses of the works of
Rosenstock[1] and Becker.[2,3] The Health Belief Model (Fig. 1) is
utilized to facilitate the understanding of the consumer's perceptions of health and illness. This model can be modified to reflect
the viewpoint of health care providers. When this is implemented,
(Fig. 2), the material provides a means of reinspecting the differences between professional and lay expectations. Thus, one may
forge a link between the two and better understand how people
perceive themselves in relation to illness and what motivates them
to seek medical help and then follow that advice.

Perceived Susceptibility

How susceptible to a certain condition does a person consider
himself to be? For example, a woman whose family does not have
a history of breast cancer is unlikely to consider herself susceptible to that disease. However, a woman whose mother and maternal
aunt both died of breast cancer may well consider herself highly
susceptible. In this case, the provider may concur with this perception of susceptibility on the basis of known "risk factors."

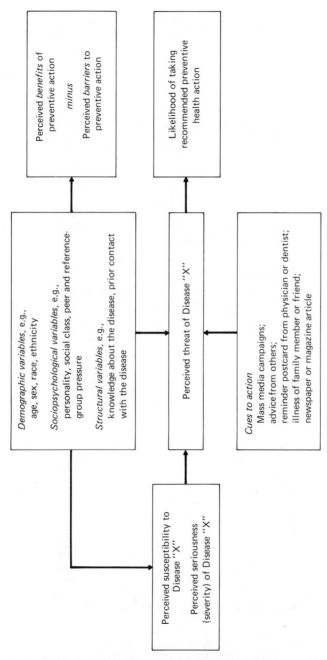

FIGURE 1. The "health-belief model" as a predictor of preventive health behavior. Reprinted with permission from M. H. Becker, R. H. Drachman, and J. T. Kirscht, "A New Approach to Explaining Sick Role Behavior in Low-income Populations," *American Journal of Public Health* 64 (1974): 206.

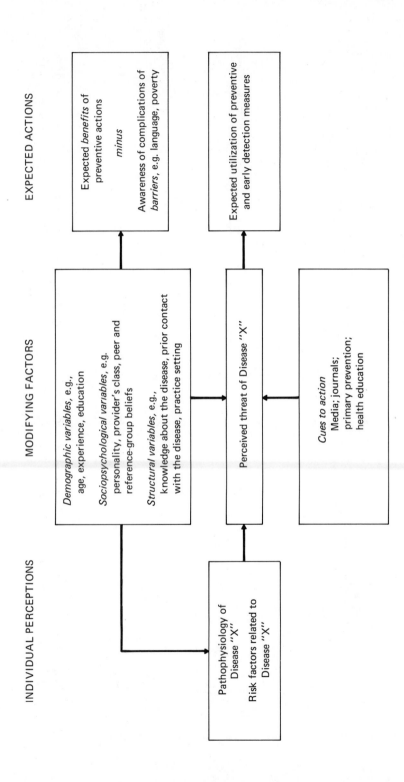

FIGURE 2.   The "health-belief model" from the provider's point of view.

Perceived Seriousness

The degree of a certain problem's seriousness varies from one person to another. It is in some measure related to the amount of difficulty that the person believes this problem will cause him. From his background in pathophysiology, the provider knows—within a certain range—how serious a problem is and may or may not withhold information from the client.

Perceived Benefits: Taking Action

What kind of action does a person take when he feels that he is susceptible to a given problem, and what are the barriers that prevent him from taking action? If a person decides that the condition is serious, he may seek help from a doctor or some other significant person, or he may vacillate and prolong the seeking and use of help for as long as possible. There are countless factors that enter into the decision-making process. Several that may act as *barriers* to care are cost, availability, and the time that will be missed from work.

From the provider's viewpoint, there is a set definition of *who* should be consulted when a given problem occurs; *when,* during that problem's course, help should be sought; and *what* therapy should be prescribed.

Modifying Factors

The *modifying factors* listed in the model are relevant because it is with respect to these factors that the areas of conflict between consumer and provider can be most readily pointed out.

Demographic Variables: Race and Ethnicity

These variables are most often cited as problem areas when the provider is white and middle class and the consumer is an ethnic person of color. This text will demonstrate the difficulty that providers have in defining health and illness, and later chapters will explore the meaning of health and illness as perceived by the ethnic person of color. Such perceptions vary not only among groups but also among individuals.

Sociopsychologic Variables

The variables of social-class, peer-, and reference-group pressures also vary between the provider and consumer and among the different ethnic groups. For example, if the consumer's belief system as to the causes of illness is "traditional" and the provider interprets etiology from a "modern" stance, there is inevitable conflict between the two viewpoints. This is even more evident when the provider is unaware of the consumer's traditional beliefs. Quite often, there are class differences between the consumer and provider: the reference group of the provider is that of the "technological health system" whereas the reference group of the consumer may well be that of the "traditional system" of health care and health-care deliverers.

Structural Variables

The structural variables also differ when the provider sees the problem from one angle and the consumer sees it from a different angle. Often, each is seeing the same thing but is using different terms (or jargon) to explain it; consequently neither is understood. Reference-group problems are also manifested in this area, and the media are an important structural variable.

Each chapter of this book represents a discrete presentation of a given topic. It in no way presents the total number of arguments or concepts relevant to a given topic. In addition, each chapter contains an annotated bibliography to assist the reader in search of further clarification of each issue.

The first unit focuses on the provider's knowing himself in terms of his perceptions and understanding of health and illness (Chapters 1 and 2). The readers are then asked to do a family history to determine what methods were practiced in their own families to prevent and treat illness. The results of what students have learned by doing this history and what it means to them are described and discussed in Chapter 3.

Unit II focuses on the broad issues of health-care delivery, culture, and healing.

It is no secret that much of the idealism that has been associated with the delivery of health care is not, in reality, justified. Yet, providers are naive in their knowledge and awareness of the harsh realities of health care. In Chapter 4, the reader is exposed to the multifaceted problems of health-care delivery and some of the more negative aspects of the system, as well as the important issue of human rights. In addition, Chapter 8 explores the dilemma of the right to health care.

The concept of culture and the role it plays in one's perception of health and illness are explored. This is first done in broad and general terms: What is culture? How is it transmitted? What is ethnicity? How does it affect a person? These and many other issues are analyzed in Chapter 5. Furthermore, the concept of culture is then taken from its broad anthropologic and sociologic definitions and brought into concrete and specific terms.

The concept of faith is also explored. It is an increasingly important issue, which is evolving to a point where the professional must have some understanding of this phenomenon. Faith plays a major role in treatment—in outcome and in success of cure. People of diverse backgrounds today acknowledge using faith healers and other types of healers. In Chapter 6 the philosophy of the holistic approach to health care is examined. A discussion of healing and alternative healers is presented.

Unit III serves as a bridge between the abstract issues and the traditional beliefs of health and illness as seen among ethnic peoples of color. Since poverty, too, plays a role in determining one's perception of and ability to cope with health and illness, Chapter 7 explores many relevant issues regarding poverty and explores the multiple ways it serves as a barrier to health and health care. Chapter 8, as earlier mentioned, explores the question "Is Health a Right?"

Once the study of each of these components has been completed, the text moves on to explore various ethnic groups in more detail. There is little doubt that these pages cannot do full justice to the richness of a health-belief system of any group of people. Nonetheless, by presenting some of the beliefs and practices and suggesting background reading, the book can begin to sensitize the reader to the unique needs of a given group of people.

The Epilogue is devoted to an overall analysis of the book's contents and how best to utilize this knowledge in health planning, health education, and health-care delivery as it relates to both the consumer and the health-care professional.

REFERENCES

1. Irwin M. Rosenstock, "Why People Use Health Services," *Millbank Memorial Fund Quarterly* 44, no. 3 (July 1966): 94-127.
2. Marshall H. Becker, et al, "A New Approach to Explaining Sick Role Behavior in Low Income Populations," *American Journal of Public Health* 64 (1974): 205-216.
3. Marshall H. Becker, *The Health Belief Model and Personal Health Behavior*. Thorofare, N.J. 1974.

BIBLIOGRAPHY: INTRODUCTION

Allport, Gordon W. *The Nature of Prejudice* (abridged). Garden City, N.Y.: Doubleday, 1958.

This book is a classic study of prejudice—the how, what, who, when, and why. Excellent background reading for study of race relations and for understanding the issues that underlie prejudice.

Jung, Carl G., editor. *Man and His Symbols*, Garden City, N.Y.: Doubleday, 1964.

Jung and others illustrate the various ways man explains his relationship to self, others, world, and nature by the use of art.

FURTHER SUGGESTED READING

Spector, Rachel E. "Health and Illness among Ethnic People of Color" *Nurse Educator* Vol. 2, no. 3 (May-June 1977): 10-16.

UNIT I
Provider
Self-Awareness

This unit enables the reader to become aware of his or her personal beliefs about health and illness. The reader is helped to:

1. Reexamine and redefine the concepts of health and illness.
2. Understand the multiple relationships between health and illness.
3. Associate the concepts of good and evil and light and dark with health and illness.
4. Trace one's own family's practices in:
   a. The protection and maintenance of health;
   b. The prevention of illness;
   c. The diagnosis and treatment of illness.
5. Understand the behavioral variances in health and illness.

6. Understand the variety of influences that one's culture and ethnicity have on the interpretations of the concepts of health and illness.

CHAPTER 1

Health

Before you begin to read this chapter, please answer the following questions:

1. How do you define health?
2. How do you keep yourself healthy?

Life is an adventure in a world where nothing is static; where unpredictable and ill-understood events constitute dangers that must be overcome, often blindly and at great cost; where man himself, like the sorcerer's apprentice, has set in motion forces that are potentially destructive and may someday escape his control. The very process of living is a continual interplay between the individual and his environment, often taking the form of a struggle resulting in injury or disease. Complete and lasting freedom from disease is but a dream remembered from imaginings of a Garden of Eden designed for the welfare of man.

—*René Dubos, Mirage of Health*

To begin our quest for a deeper understanding of the problems surrounding the delivery of adequate health care, let us ask: "What is health?" One response may be flawless recitation of the standard definition of the World Health Organization (WHO), given with great assurance—a challenge neither expected nor welcomed, and probably evoking an intense dispute wherein an assumed right answer is completely torn apart. Answers such as "homeostasis," "kinetic energy in balance," "optimal functioning," and "freedom from pain" are opened to discussion. Experienced health-care providers may be unable to give a comprehensive, acceptable answer to such a seemingly simple question. It is difficult to give a definition that makes sense without the use of some form of medical jargon. It is also challenging to articulate a clear meaning in terms that a lay person could understand. (We lack skill in understanding "health" in the layman's perspective.)

A basic example of the many and varying definitions is in the *American Heritage Dictionary:*

> n. 1. The state of an organism with respect to functioning, disease, and abnormality at any given time. 2. The state of an organism functioning normally without disease or abnormality. 3. Optimal functioning with freedom from disease and abnormality. 4. Broadly, any state of optimal functioning, well being, or progress. 5. A wish for someone's good health, expressed as a toast.[1]

Murray and Zentner define health as "a purposeful, adaptive response, physically, mentally, emotionally and socially, to internal and external stimuli in order to maintain stability and comfort."[2] The WHO defines health as a "state of complete physical, mental, and social well being and not merely the absence of disease."

These definitions—each unique and varying in scope and context—are essentially the definitions that the student, practitioner, and educator within the health professions agree convey the meaning of health. The most widely utilized and recognized definition is that of WHO. Within the socialization process of the health-care deliverer the connotation of the word is that contained in the WHO definition; for other students the word becomes clear through the educational experience.

In analyzing these definitions, one is able to discern subtle variations in denotation. If this occurs in the denotation of the word, what of the connotation? That is, are health-care providers as familiar with implicit meanings as with those that are more explicit? If the following comment (made in a discussion of an article by Irwin M. Rosenstock) is accurate, then the educational process is indeed deficient:

> Whereas health itself is in reality an elusive concept, in much of research, the stages involved in seeking medical care are conceived as completely distinct. The health professions are becoming increasingly aware of the *lack of clarity* in the definition of health.[3]

However, the framework of both education and research in the health professions continues to utilize the more abstract definitions of the word "health." When the broader connotations are considered, one can conceive that health is regarded not only as the absence of disease but also as a reward for "good behavior." In fact, a state of health is regarded by many peoples as the reward one receives for "good" behavior or a punishment for "bad" behavior. Frequently people state, "She is so good; no wonder she is so healthy." The mother admonishes the child, "If you don't do such and such, you'll get sick." There are countless situations and experiences that are avoided for the purpose of protecting and maintaining one's health. Quite often, people seek challenges. In some instances individuals seek out challenging, albeit dangerous, situations with the hope that they will experience the thrill of a challenge and still emerge in an intact state of health. One example of this is driving at high speeds.

There is also the viewpoint that health is the freedom from and the absence of evil. In this context, health is analogous to day, which equals good, which equals light. Conversely, illness is analogous to night, which equals evil, which equals dark. Illness, to some, is seen as a punishment for being bad or doing evil deeds; it is the work of vindictive evil spirits. In the "modern" education of health-care providers, these concepts of health and illness are rarely, if ever, discussed. Yet it can be maintained that—if these concepts of health and illness are believed by people within the general population, including consumers of health-care services— then understanding these varying ideas is vital to enabling the provider to comprehend the beliefs of consumers with whom they come in contact.

We each enter the health-care community with a unique, culturally based concept of health. During the educational and socialization process in our given profession—be it nursing, medicine, or social work—we are expected to shed these beliefs and adopt the aforementioned definitions. In addition to shedding these old beliefs, we learn, if only by unspoken example, to view as deviant those who do not accept the prevailing, institutional connotation of the word "health."

The material that follows illustrates the complex process necessary to enable providers to return to and appreciate their former interpretations of health, to understand the vast number of meanings the word health has, and to be aware of the difficulties that exist with definitions such as that of the World Health Organization.

HOW DO YOU DEFINE HEALTH?

You have been requested to describe the term *health* in your own words. An initial response to this request is frequently a recital of the WHO definition. What does this definition really mean? The following is a representative sample of responses:

1. Being able to do what I want to do.
2. Physical and psychological well-being, *physical* meaning

that there are no abnormal functions with the body, all systems are without those abnormal functions that would cause a problem physically, and *psychological* meaning that one's mind is capable of a clear and logical thinking process and association.

3. Being able to use all of your body parts in the way that you want to—to have energy and enthusiasm.
4. Being able to perform your normal activities, such as working, without discomfort and at an optimal level.
5. The state of wellness with no physical or mental illness.
6. I would define health as an undefined term. It depends on the situations, individuals, and other things.

In the initial step of the "unlocking" process,* it begins to become clear that there is not a set rule that states what health really is. We can all agree on the United Nations definition, but when asked "What does that mean?" we are unable to clarify further, or to simplify that definition. As we begin to perceive a change in the connotation of the word, we may experience dismay that an emotional response often accompanies the breaking down of ideas. When this occurs, we begin to realize that as we were socialized into the provider culture, via the educational process, our understanding of health changed and we moved a great distance from our older understanding of the term. The following list includes the definitions of health given by students in various levels of their education and experiences. The students ranged in age from 19-year-old college juniors to adult nursing trainees and graduate students in both nuring and social work.

Junior students: A system involving all subsystems of one's body that constantly work on keeping one in physical and mental condition.

Senior students: Ability to function in activities of daily living to optimal capacity without requiring medical attention.
Mental and physical wellness.
The state of physical, mental, and emotional well-being.

*The "unlocking" process includes those steps taken to help break down and understand the definitions of both *health* and *illness* in a "living" context. It consists of persistent questioning: "What is Health?" must be asked over and over again. No matter what the response, the question "What does that mean?" is asked. Initially, this causes much confusion, but in classroom practice—as each term is written on the blackboard and analyzed—the air clears and the process begins to make sense.

RN students: Ability to cope with stressors.
Absence of pain—mental and physical.
State of optimal well-being, both physically and emotionally.

Graduate students: State of well-being that is free from physical and mental distress. I can also include in this social well-being, even though this may be idealistic.
Not only the absence of disease, but a state of balance or equilibrium among physical, emotional, and spiritual states of well-being.

It appears that the definition becomes more abstract and technical as the student advances in the educational program. The terms utilized to explain health take on a more abstract and scientific character with each year of removal from the lay way of thinking.

The problem now arises as to how these layers of jargon can be removed and whether it is possible to help ourselves once again to view health in a more tangible manner.

The next step in probing this matter is to think back to the way we perceived health before our entrance into the educational program. I believe that the farther back one can go in his memory of earlier concepts of health, the better. Again, the question "What is health?" is asked over and over. Initially, the responses continue to include such terms and phrases as "homeostasis," "freedom from disease," or "frame of mind." Slowly, and with considerable prodding, we are able to recall earlier perceptions of health: once again, health becomes a *personal, experiential* concept, and the relation of *health* to *being* returns. The fragility and instability of this concept are also recognized as the term gradually becomes a meaningful concept in relation to *being*.

This process of unlocking a perception of a concept takes a considerable amount of time and patience. It also engenders dismay that briefly turns to anger and resentment. One may question why the definitions acquired and mastered in the learning process are now being challenged and torn apart. The feeling may be that of taking a giant step backward in a quest for new terminology and new knowledge.

Yet with this unlocking process, one is able to perceive the concept of health *in the way that a vast number of health-care consumers may perceive it*. The following illustrates the transition that the concept passed through in an "unlocking process" from the WHO definition to the realm of the health-care consumer:

> *Initial responses*:   Feeling of well-being, no illness.
> Homeostasis.
> Complete physical, mental, and social well-being.
>
> *Secondary responses*:   Frame of mind.
> Subjective state of psychosocial well-being.
> Activities of daily living can be performed.
>
> *Experiential responses*:   (Health becomes tangible; the description is articulated by using qualities that can be seen, felt, or touched.)
> Shiny hair.
> Warm, smooth, glossy skin.
> Clear eyes.
> Shiny teeth.
> Being alert.
> Being happy.
> Freedom from pain.
> Harmony between body and mind.

Yet, even this itemized description does not completely answer the question, "What is health?" The words are once again subjected to the question, "What does that mean?" and once again the terms are stripped down and a paradox begins to emerge. For example, it is pointed out that "shiny hair" may in fact be present in an ill person or in a person who has not washed his hair for a long period of time. In the healthy person, clean, well-groomed hair with lustre may not always be present.

It becomes clear that no matter how much one goes around in a circle in an attempt to define "health" clearly, the terms and meanings attributed to the state can be challenged. The result of this prolonged discussion is that one never really comes to an acceptable definition of health. Yet, by going through the intense "unlocking" process, one is able finally to understand the vast amount of difficulty that surrounds the word. In a highly personal manner we are now sensitized to variations in the meanings of the word *health* and its many definitions. Thus we are less likely to view as deviant those people who have other beliefs and practices in relation to their own health and health care.

Preventive Care and Health Maintenance

It has been suggested in the preceding material that there are multiple ways of viewing health. It has been demonstrated that there are many areas of disagreement with respect to how this word can be defined. "Health is not merely an end in itself, but rather a means of attaining human well-being within the natural constraints in which man finds himself."[4] To state it another way:

> ... any aspect of health for an individual, or the determiners of what he does or does not do in relation to some aspect of health, is some combination of the effects of his physical body: what he knows about it, what he feels about it, and how significant others react to it.[5]

The preparation of health-care workers tends to structure education from an illness perspective; rarely (or superficially) does it include a study of the concept of *health*. Today, however, the emphasis is shifting from acute care to preventive care. The need for the provider of health services to comprehend this concept is, therefore, crucial. If this movement for preventive health care is to take hold, become firmly entrenched, and thrive, there are multiple issues that must be resolved in answering the question: "What is health?" Unless the provider is able to understand health from the viewpoint of the consumer, a barrier of misunderstanding grows and is perpetuated. It is a difficult process to reexamine complex definitions dutifully memorized at an earlier time. Yet an understanding of health from a client's viewpoint is essential to the establishment of preventive health-care services because the perception of health is a complex psychological process. It is selective in that "man sees what he wants to see or expects to see."[6] There tends to be no established pattern in what individuals and families see as their health needs and how they go about practicing their own health care.[7] Yet their perception of health is sanctioned and given meaning when it is brought to a level of awareness where it can be interpreted and used in planning the future.[8]

Health maintenance and the prevention of illness are by no means new concepts. As long as human beings have existed, they have used a multitude of methods—ranging from magic and witchcraft to present-day immunization—in an ongoing effort to maintain good health and prevent debilitating illness. Raquel Cohen sees prevention as "a plea for early intervention to help people deal more successfully with the difficulties arising from man's struggles to adapt to society."[9] Another current viewpoint regarding prevention is advanced by Richard Stark: "Health maintenance has become our national obsession. Logic suggests that in order to maintain health we must prevent disease, and that is best accomplished by eating balanced meals, exercising regularly, and seeing the doctor once a year for a checkup."[10] The annual ritual of visiting a physician has been extensively promoted by the medical establishment and is viewed as effective by numerous lay people. A doctor's statement is often required by a person seeking employment and/or life insurance.[11] Furthermore, the annual physical examination has been advertised as the key to good health. A "clean bill of health" is considered essential for social, emotional, and even economic success. This clean bill of health is bestowed only by the members of the medical profession. The general public has been conditioned to believe that health is guaranteed if a disease that may be developing is discovered early and treated with the ever-increasing modalities of modern medical technology.[12] Yet for all those who believe in and practice the ritual of the annual physical and screening for early detection of a disease, there are those—both within and outside of the health-care professions—who do not subscribe to the annual ritual of the physical examination.[13] Preventive medicine grew out of clinical practice associated either with welfare medicine or with industrial or occupational medical practice. The approach of preventive medicine and health maintenance is now developing as a new focus for health-care practice in the United States.[14]

Health Diaries

Keeping a 30-day health diary is recommended to increase awareness of one's own health status and health practices. If an illness occurs, record what is done for it, why it is done, and what type of health-care services was utilized.

Comments will be most revealing! We recognize that, in spite of the fact that we are learning "proper" methods of health maintenance, we have poor nutritional and sleeping habits and rarely, if ever, seek medical help for what some of us consider "serious" bodily complaints. At best, seeking care is delayed until we give up the idea that our symptoms will disappear. This diary has a very sobering effect. It is also used as an additional "humanizing" tool. The word *humanizing* is used here because just as we treat ourselves and/or delay in seeking help, we ought not judge people who, for various reasons, also treat themselves and/or delay in seeking health care.

The following exercise is designed to help the reader "tune in" to his own daily health status.

Keep a daily record of your health status and behavior for 30 days. Include in this record medications taken (prescription and nonprescription), eating, sleeping, exercise, and recreational activities. When appropriate, note the reasons for your actions.

The daily record, or diary, enables you to see how you react to the various stresses and strains of daily life. It reveals the intricacies of your daily lifestyle—the things you take for granted. For example: Do you eat three balanced meals a day? Do you get enough rest? Do you exercise?

At the end of 30 days reread this diary and analyze it in relation to recommended health practices.

Typical entries for such a record follow.

Monday	overslept (went to bed 3:00 A.M.)
	skipped breakfast
	dozed in class
	coke and cheese crackers for lunch
	2 aspirins (headache)
	hamburger and french fries for supper
	crashed at 8:00 P.M.
Tuesday	up at 6:30 for clinical
	milk and toast for breakfast
	exercise—walk in hospital corridors
	supper—lasagne, wine
	headache—2 aspirins
	bed 8:00 P.M. (couldn't study)
Wednesday	up at 7:00 for 8:30 lecture
	walked to hospital
	no breakfast (not hungry)
	peanut butter & jelly for lunch
	P.M. snack—milk & candy bar

<pre>
                    study until 2:00 A.M.
                    2 aspirins (headache)
    Thursday   up at 6:30 for clinical
                    coffee and cheese sandwich for breakfast
                    walked to hospital (it rained)
                    almost slept on ward
                    no lunch (out of funds—no time to cash
                       check)
                    coke
                    walked in hospital corridors
</pre>

In summary, this chapter has attempted to deal solely with the concept of *health*. The multiple denotations and connotations of the word have been explored. A method for helping you to "tune in" to your health has been included.

REFERENCES

1. *American Heritage Dictionary of the English Language,* s.v. "health."
2. Ruth Murray and Judith Zentner, *Nursing Concepts for Health Promotion* (Englewood Cliffs, N.J.: Prentice-Hall, 1975), p. 6.
3. Discussion of article by Irwin M. Rosenstock, "Why People Use Health Services," *Milbank Memorial Fund Quarterly* 44, no. 3 (July 1966): 94-127.
4. Herman E. Hilleboe, "Preventing Future Shock: Health Developments in the 1960's and Imperative for the 1970's," *American Journal of Public Health*, February 1972, p. 139.
5. Robert D. Russell, "Teaching for Meaning in Health Education: The Concept Approach," *Journal of School Health* 71 (January 1966): 13-14.
6. Francis L. Harmon, *Principles of Psychology* (Milwaukee: University of Wisconsin Press, 1951), p. 14; William N. Dember, *The Psychology of Perception* (New York: Holt, 1960), pp. 3-4.
7. Alexander A. Schneiders, *Introductory Psychology* (New York: Rinehart, 1960), p. 185.
8. Andiel Knutson, *The Individual, Society, and Health Behavior* (New York: Russell Sage Foundation, 1965), p. 159.
9. Raquel Cohen, "Principles of Preventive Mental Health Programs for Ethnic Minority Populations," *American Journal of Psychiatry* 128, no. 12 (June 1972): 1531.
10. Richard Stark, "The Case Against Regular Physicals," *New York Times Magazine*, (25 July 1976), p. 10.
11. Stephen B. Yohalen, *New York Times Magazine* (15 August, 1976), p. 58.

12. Manuel Spector and Rachel Spector, "Is Prevention Myth or Reality?" *Health Education* 8, no. 4 (July-August 1977): 23-26.

13. Ibid.

14. John G. Freymann, "Medicine's Great Schism: Prevention vs. Cure," *Medical Care* 12, no. 7 (July 1975): 533.

CHAPTER 2

Illness

Before you begin to read this chapter, please answer the following questions:

1. How do *you* define illness?
2. What would you define as a minor or "not serious" medical problem? Give examples.
3. How do you know when a given health problem does not need medical attention?
4. Do you "self-diagnose" when a health problem presents itself? Give examples.
5. Do you use over-the-counter medications? Which ones and when?

The world of illness is the one that is most familiar to the nurse and other providers of health care. It is in this world that the provider feels most comfortable and useful.

There are many questions to be answered: What determines illness? How does an individual know when he is ill? What provokes a person to seek help from the health-care system? At what point is health care sought when an individual or his significant others determine he can no longer treat the disorder himself? Where does a person go for help? To whom does he go for help?

We tend to regard illness as the absence of health, yet it has been demonstrated in the preceding chapter that *health* is at best an elusive term that defies a specific definition! Let us look at the present issue more closely. Is illness the opposite of health? Is it a permanent condition or a transient condition? How does one know that he is ill?

The *American Heritage Dictionary* defines "illness" as "Sickness of body or mind. b. sickness. 2. *obsolete.* Evil; wickedness."[1]

As with *health,* the word *illness* can be subjected to extensive analysis. What is illness? For example, a generalized response, such as "abnormal functioning of a body's system or systems," evolves into more specific assessments of what we observe and believe to be wrong. Thus illness is a "sore throat," a "headache," or a "fever"—the latter determined not necessarily by the measurement on a thermometer, but by the flushed face; the warm-to-hot feeling of the forehead, back, and abdomen; and the overall malaise that such an individual tends to experience. To clarify this concept further, the diagnosis of "intestinal obstruction," for example, becomes described as pain in the stomach (really the abdomen, but lay people call it stomach), which is worse than that caused by "gas," as well as severe upset stomach, nausea, vomiting, and marked constipation.

Essentially, we are being pulled back in the popular direction and encouraged to reuse lay terms. We initially resist this because we want to utilize professional jargon. (Why reuse lay terms when our knowledge is so much greater?) It is crucial that we be called to task for using jargon; we must learn to be constantly conscious of the way in which the laity perceives illness and health care.

Another factor emerges as the word illness is stripped down

to its barest essentials. Many of the characteristics attributed to health occur in illness, too. A rude awakening or "reality shock" comes about when one realizes that a person perceived as healthy by clinical assessment may then—by a given set of symptoms—define himself as ill (or vice versa). For example, in summertime one may see a person with a red face and assume that he has a sunburn. The person may, in fact, have a fever. A person recently discharged from the hospital, pale and barely able to walk, may be judged ill. However, that individual may consider himself *well* because he is much better than when he entered the hospital—now he is able to walk! Thus perceptions are relative, and, in this instance, the eyes of the beholder have been befuddled by inadequate information and input. Unfortunately, at the provider's level of practice, we do not always ask the person: "How do you view your state of health?" Rather, we determine his state of health on objective and observational data.

As is the case with the concept of health, one learns in nursing or medical school how to determine what illness is and how people are expected to behave when they are ill. Yet once these terms are separated and examined, the models that health-care providers have created tend to carry little weight. There is little agreement as to what specifically illness is. Yet, in view of the contradictions inherent in the answers, one nonetheless has a high level of expectation as to what behavior should be demonstrated by both the client and provider when illness occurs! One discovers that we have a vast amount of knowledge with respect to the acute illnesses and the services that must ideally be provided for the acutely ill person. However, when the contradictions surface, one finds that one has minimal knowledge of the vast "gray" area: e.g., whether someone is questionably ill, or becoming ill with what may later be an acute episode. Because of the ease with which one often identifies cardinal symptoms, one finds that he is able to react to acute illness and may have negative attitudes toward those who do not seek help when the first symptom of an acute illness appears. The questions that then arise are: What is an acute illness, and how does one differentiate between it and some everyday indisposition that most people treat by themselves? When does one draw the line and admit that the disorder is out of the realm of adequate self-treatment?

These are certainly very difficult questions to answer, especially when careful analysis shows that even the parameters of an acute illness tend to vary from one person to another! In many acute illnesses, the symptoms are so severe that the person experiencing them has little choice but to seek immediate medical care. Such is the case with a severe myocardial infarction. But what about the person who experiences mild discomfort in the epigastric region? He might say, "I have indigestion," and self-medicate with baking soda, an antacid, milk, or Alka Seltzer. Even if he experiences mild pain in the left arm he may delay in seeking care because he believes that the pain will disappear. Obviously, this person may be as ill, if not more so, than the person who seeks help during the onset of symptoms, but he will, like most people, minimize these small aches because—for many different reasons—he may not want to assume the sick role.

THE SICK ROLE

In order to help explain the phenomenon of "the sick role," the work of Talcott Parsons is utilized. In our society, a person is expected to have the symptoms that he views as illness confirmed as such by a member of the health-care profession. In other words, the sick role must first be legitimately conferred on him by the keepers of this privilege: a person cannot legitimize his own illness and have his own diagnosis accepted by the society at large. Hence "a legitimate procedure for the definition and sanctioning of the adoption of the sick role is fundamental for both the social system and the sick individual."[2]

Role is defined sociologically (1) as the set of expectations and behaviors associated with a specific position in a social system (social role) or (2) as the way an individual personality tends to react to a social situation (individual role).[3] Illness "is not merely a 'condition' but also a social role."[4] There are four main components inherent in the sick role:

1. "The sick person is exempted from the performance of certain of his/her normal social obligations."[5] An example is a student nurse who has a

severe sore throat and decides that she does not want to go to her clinical assignment. In order for her to be exempted from the day's activities, she must have this symptom validated by someone in the health services, either a physician or the nurse on duty. Her claim of illness must be legitimized or socially defined and validated by a sanctioned provider of health-care services.

2. "The sick person is also exempted from a certain type of responsibility for his/her own state."[6] For example, when a person becomes ill, he cannot be expected to "pull himself together" or to be spontaneously cured. The student with the sore throat is expected to seek help and then to follow the advice of the attending physician or nurse in helping her to recover. The student is not responsible for her recovery except in a peripheral sense.

3. "The legitimization of the sick role is, however, only partial".[7] When one is "sick," he is in an undesirable state and *should* recover and leave this state as rapidly as possible. The student's sore throat is acceptable only for a while; beyond a reasonable amount of time—as determined by the physician, his peers, and the faculty—she can no longer claim legitimate absence from the clinical classroom setting.

4. "Being sick, except in the mildest of cases, is being in need of help."[8] The type of help, as defined by the majority sector of American society and other Western countries, is that of the physician. In seeking the help of the physician, the person now not only bears the sick role but in addition takes on the role of patient. Patienthood carries with it a certain prescribed set of responsibilities, some of which include compliance with a medical regimen, cooperation with the health-care provider, and following orders without asking too many questions. All of this leads to the illness experience, which we will discuss below.

THE ILLNESS EXPERIENCE

The experience of an illness is determined by what illness means to the sick person. Furthermore, illness refers to a specific status and role within a given society. Not only must illness be sanctioned by a physician in order for the sick person to assume the sick role, but it must also be sanctioned by the community or social structure of which the person is a member. This experience can be divided into four stages that are sufficiently general to cover the interpretation of a given problem within any society or culture.

Onset

"Onset" is when the person experiences the first symptoms of a given problem.[9] This event can be slow and insidious or rapid and acute. When the onset is insidious, the patient may not be conscious of symptoms, or may think that if he waits the discomfort will go away. If, on the other hand, the onset is acute, the person is positive that he is ill and knows that he must seek immediate help. "This stage is seen as the prelude to legitimization of illness."[10]

Diagnosis

In this stage of the illness experience, the disease is identified or an effort is made to identify it.[11] The individual is now sanctioned in his role, and at this point the illness is socially recognized and identified. At this point the health-care providers make decisions pertaining to appropriate therapy. During the period of diagnosis, the person experiences another phenomenon: dealing with the unknown, which includes fearing what the diagnosis will be.

For many people, going through a medical work-up is an unfamiliar experience. This is made doubly difficult because they are asked and expected to relate to strange people who are doing unfamiliar and often painful things to their bodies and minds. To the lay person, the environment of the hospital and/or physician's office is both strange and unfamiliar, and it is natural to fear these qualities. Quite often, the ailing individual is faced with a diagnosis that he knows nothing about. Nonetheless, he is expected to follow closely a prescribed treatment plan that is usually detailed to him by the health-care providers, but which in all likelihood may not accommodate his unique life-style. The situation is that of a horizontal-vertical dichotomy: the patient being figuratively and literally in the former position, the professional in the latter.

Patient Status

During this period the person adjusts to the "social aspects of being ill and gives in to the demands of his/her physical condition."[12] The sick role becomes that of patienthood, and the person is expected to shift into this role as society determines it should be enacted. The person must make any necessary alterations in his life-style, become dependent on others in some circumstances for the basic needs of daily life, and adapt to the demands of his physical condition as well as to treatment limitations and expectations. The environment of the patient is highly structured. The parameters of his world are determined by the providers of the health-care services, not by the patient. Therein lies the conflict.

There has been much written describing the environment of the hospital and the roles that people in such an institution play. As was stated, the hospital is typically unfamiliar to the patient, yet he is expected to conform to a predetermined set of rules and behaviors, many of which are unwritten and undefined for him— let alone *by* him.

Recovery

The final stage is "generally characterized by the relinquishing of patient status and the assumption of pre-patient roles and activities."[13] There is often a change in the roles a person is able to play and the activities he is able to perform once recovery takes

---

Table 1. A Tool for the Assessment of

Onset	Diagnosis

A. The Meaning of the Illness

1. What symptoms does this patient complain of?
2. How does he judge the extent and kind of disease?
3. How does this illness fit with his image of health? Himself?
4. How does the disease threaten him?
5. Why did he seek medical help?

1. Does he understand the diagnosis?
2. How does he interpret the illness?
3. How can he adapt to the illness?
4. How does he think others feel about it?

B. Behavior in Response to Illness

1. How does he control anxiety?
2. How are affective responses to concerns expressed?
3. Did he seek some form of health care before he sought medical care?

1. What treatment agents were used?

Adapted from Alksne et al.[14]

place. Often recovery is not complete. The person may be left with an undesirable or unexpected change in his body image or in his ability to perform expected or routine everyday activities. One example might be that of a woman who enters the hospital with a small lump in her breast and who, after having surgery, subsequently returns home with only one breast. Another example: a laborer who enters the hospital with a backache and returns home after a laminectomy; when he returns to work, he cannot reassume his position as a loader. Obviously, an entire life-style must be altered to accommodate such newly imposed changes.

the Patient During the Four Stages of Illness

Patient Status	Recovery
1. Has his perception of the illness changed? 2. What are the changes in his life as a consequence of it? 3. What is his goal in recovery—the same level of health as before the illness, attainment of a maximal level of wellness, or perfect health? 4. How does he relate to medical professionals? 5. What are his social pressures leading to recovery? 6. What is motivating him to recover?	1. What are signs of recovery? 2. Can he reassume his prepatient role and functions? 3. Has his self-image been changed? 4. How does he see his present state of health—as more vulnerable or resistant?
1. How does he handle the patient role? 2. How does he relate to the medical personnel?	1. Are there any permanent after-effects from this illness? 2. How does he reassume his old role?

From the viewpoint of the provider, such an individual has recovered: his body no longer has the symptoms of the acute illness that made surgical treatment necessary. Yet, in the eyes of the patient, he is still sick because he can no longer do what he is accustomed to doing. So many changes have been wrought that it is no wonder if he seems perplexed and/or uncooperative. Here, too, there is certainly conflict between society's expectations and the person's expectation. Society releases him from the sick role at a time when, subjectively, he may not be ready to relinquish it.

Table 1 is a tool designed for the assessment of the patient during the four stages of illness. Originally designed as a sociologic measuring tool, the material has been altered here to meet the needs of the health-care provider in achieving better understanding of patient behavior and expectations. If the provider is able to obtain answers from the patient to all of the questions raised in the tool, he will be able to understand the patient's behavior and perspective and subsequently attempt to provide safe, effective care.

Another method of dividing the illness experience into stages was developed by the late Dr. Edward A. Suchman. He divided the experience into five components entitled exactly as are the subheadings that follow.

The Symptom Experience Stage

The person is physically and cognitively aware that something is wrong, and he responds emotionally.[15]

The Assumption of the Sick Role Stage

The person seeks help and shares his problem with family and friends. He moves through the lay referral system, seeking advice, reassurance, and validation. He is temporarily excused from various responsibilities such as work, school, and other activities of daily living as his condition dictates.[16]

The Medical Care Contact Stage

At this time the person seeks out the "scientific" rather than the "lay" diagnosis. He wants to know: "Am I really sick?" "What is wrong with me?" "What does it mean?" It is at this point that the sick person needs some knowledge of the health-care system, what the system offers, and how it functions. This knowledge assists him in selecting the resources that he utilizes and in interpreting the information that he receives.[17]

The Dependent-Patient Role Stage

The patient is now under the control of the physician and is expected to accept and comply with the prescribed treatments. The person may be quite ambivalent about this role, and certain factors (namely physical, administrative, social, or psychological) may create barriers that will eventually interfere with his treatment and his willingness to comply.[18]

The Recovery or Rehabilitation Stage

The role of patient is at this stage given up, and the person resumes—as much as possible—his former roles.[19]

SUMMARY

The purpose of this chapter has been to introduce the reader to the concept of illness, as explored from the pure act of definition and broadened through the sociological aspects of roles and behaviors. The writings of a number of sociologists have been examined in terms of applicability to nursing practice, observation, and experience.

REFERENCES

1. *American Heritage Dictionary of the English Language*, s.v. "illness."
2. David Mechanic, *Medical Sociology* (New York: Free Press of Glencoe, 1968), p. 80.
3. David Popenoe, *Sociology* (New York: Appleton, 1974), p. 681.
4. Talcott Parsons, "Illness and the Role of the Physician: A Sociological Perspective," in *Medical Care: Readings in the Sociology of Medical Institutions*, W. Richard Scott and Edmund H. Volkart, editors (New York: Wiley, 1966), p. 275.
5. Ibid.
6. Ibid.
7. Ibid.
8. Ibid., p. 276.
9. Lois Alksne et al., *"A Conceptual Framework for the Analysis of Cultural Variations in the Behavior of the Ill"* (unpublished, undated report, New York City Department of Health), p. 2.

10. Ibid., p. 3.
11. Ibid.
12. Ibid.
13. Ibid.
14. Lois Alksne et al., op. cit.
15. Edward A. Suchman, "Stages of Illness and Medical Care," *Journal of Health and Human Behavior* 6, 3 (Fall 1965): 114.
16. Ibid., p. 115.
17. Ibid.
18. Ibid.
19. Ibid., p. 116.

BIBLIOGRAPHY: HEALTH AND ILLNESS

Apple, Dorion, editor. *Sociological Studies of Health and Sickness: A Source Book for the Health Professions.* New York: McGraw-Hill, 1960.

> This anthology covers such areas as the recognition of the need for health care, the patient's viewpoint, psychosocial process in illness, and the organization of hospitals. The essays address such broad questions as "Should I have a check-up?" "What occurs when patient and physician misunderstand each other?" "What are the psychosocial determinants of illness?" and "What is the social organization of hospitals?"

Bakan, David. *Disease, Pain and Sacrifice: Toward a Psychology of Suffering.* Chicago: University of Chicago Press, 1968.

> Bakan explores the conviction that amelioration of suffering through understanding is the superior option. He describes the aspects of suffering from biological, psychological, and existential standpoints. Very highly recommended.

Becker, Marshall H. *The Health Belief Model and Personal Health Behavior.* Thorofare, N.J.: 1974.

> This monograph traces the history of the health belief model and its various uses in explaining and understanding health behavior in both health and illness.

Dubos, René Jules. *Man Adapting.* New Haven, Conn.: Yale University Press, 1965.
——. *Man, Medicine and Environment.* New York: Praeger, 1968.
——. *Mirage of Health.* Garden City, N.Y.: (Doubleday) Anchor Books, 1961.

> In these three books Dubos analyzes various aspects of human beings and their relationship to the environment. He does not explore wonder drugs but rather the wonders of life.

Freeman, Howard; Levin, Sol; and Reeder, Leo G., editors. *Handbook of Medical Sociology*, 2nd ed. Englewood Cliffs, N.J.: Prentice-Hall, 1972.

> This handbook helps to bridge the knowledge gap that exists between the biologic and social sciences. It explores such areas as the sociology of illness; practitioners, patients, and medical settings; the sociology of medical care; and the strategy, method, and status of medical sociology.

Herzlich, Claudine. *Health and Illness: A Social Psychological Analysis.* Translated by Douglas Graham. New York: Academic Press, 1973.

> Herzlich reports findings based on a study conducted in France in the 1960s: an exploration of people's attitudes toward health and illness. It investigates topics such as the individual, his way of life, and the genesis of illness; nature, constraint, and society; mechanisms and dosage; health and illness; the dimensions and limits of illness; the sick and the healthy; and health and illness behavior.

Jackson, Robert C., and Morton, Jean. *Family Health Care: Health Promotion and Illness Care.* Based on the proceedings of the 1975 Annual Insitute for Public Health Social Workers, University of California, Berkeley.

> In this work, attention is given to the broad topics of perspectives of health services to the family, strategies for the promotion of health and family functioning, and family-focused care for the ill.

Jaco, E. Gartly, editor. *Patients, Physicians, and Illness: Sourcebook in Behavioral Science and Medicine.* Glencoe, Ill. Free Press, 1958.

> This anthology is a sourcebook in behavioral science and medicine. It covers a wide range of topics including social and personal components of illness and health; community and sociocultural aspects of medical care and treatment; and the patient. Authors include Lyle Saunders, Talcott Parsons, and Mark Zborowski.

Kiev, Ari, editor. *Magic, Faith and Healing: Studies in Primitive Psychiatry Today.* New York: Free Press of Glencoe, 1964.

> Another anthology, Kiev's book explores the wide number of abnormal states of mood, thought, and behavior and the multitude of "folk" ways that are employed throughout the world to treat disorders.

Knutson, Andie L. *The Individual, Society and Health Behavior.* New York: Russell Sage Foundation, 1965.

> Herein human beings are dealt with as members of society;

emphasis is placed on those aspects of their behavior that are of concern to public health. It covers a broad range of topics, including the general characteristics of humankind; men and women in their social environment; values, attitudes, and beliefs; and the communication process.

Leff, S., and Leff, Vera. *From Witchcraft to World Health.* New York: Macmillan, 1957.

Leff and Leff report on a battle that is fought to save lives. The book relates the history of public health from the medicine man to WHO. It covers such topics as primitive man and Egyptian, Greek, and Roman medicine, and follows the development of public health through the twentieth century.

Lynch, L. Reddick, editor. *The Cross-Cultural Approach to Health Behavior.* Rutherford, N.J.: Fairleigh Dickenson University Press, 1969.

This book explores the interrelationships between sociocultural background and health behavior. The articles that are included investigate the values and beliefs about health of many people through the United States and the world.

Mechanic, David. *Medical Sociology: A Selective View.* New York: Free Press of Glencoe, 1968.

Three major sections comprise this book. The first section substantively develops a view of illness as part of the larger social interest and deviant behavior. The second explores such issues as the factors that affect mortality and morbidity. The third analyzes the various organizational contexts of practitioner-patient interactions.

Opler, Marvin K., editor. *Culture and Mental Health.* New York: Macmillan, 1959.

This anthology on social psychiatry demonstrates ways in which cultural patterns affect mental health in a worldwide perspective. Opler includes papers from every continent where work has been done.

Paul, Benjamin, editor. *Health, Culture, and Community: Case Studies of Public Reactions to Health Programs.* New York: Russell Sage Foundation, 1955.

Numerous case studies of public reactions to health programs are reported in this anthology. The cases demonstrate to health workers the kind of working relationship that ought to exist between the providers of health care and social scientists.

Pearsall, Marion. *Medical Behavioral Science: A Selected Bibliography of Cultural Anthropology, Social Psychology, and Sociology in Medicine.* Louisville: University of Kentucky Press, 1963.

An outstanding bibliography of books published through 1962 that relate to health care practices via cultural anthropology, social psychology, and sociology.

Popenoe, Cris. *Wellness.* Washington, D.C.: YES! Inc., 1977.

This book is an annotated bibliography that contains numerous books relevant to health. A sample of topics that are presented includes anatomy and physiology, body work, cooking, healing, and use of herbs. Good reference.

FURTHER SUGGESTED READINGS

Books

Alksne, L., Wellin, E., Suchman, E., and Patrick, S. *A Conceptual Framework for the Analysis of Cultural Variations in the Behavior of the Ill.* Unpublished, undated report—New York City Department of Health.

Blum, Henrick L. *Expanding Health Care Horizons.* Oakland, Calif.: Third Party Associates, 1976.

Cannon, Walter B. *The Wisdom of the Body.* New York: Norton, 1939.

Carlson, Rick J. *The End of Medicine.* New York: Wiley, 1975.

Dember, William N. *The Psychology of Perception.* New York: Holt, 1960.

Dubos, René. *Man, Medicine and Environment.* New York: Mentor, 1968.

_____. *Beast or Angel? Choices that Make us Human.* New York: Scribners, 1974.

Harmon, Frances L. *Principles of Psychology.* Madison: University of Wisconsin Press, 1951.

Murray, Ruth, and Zentner, Judith. *Nursing Concepts for Health Promotion.* Englewood Cliffs, N.J.: Prentice-Hall, 1975.

Popenoe, David. *Sociology.* New York: Appleton, 1974.

Schneiders, Alexander A. *Introduction to Psychology.* New York: Rinehart, 1960.

White, Kerr L., editor. *Life and Death and Medicine.* San Francisco: Freeman, 1973.

Articles

Becker, M. H., et al., "A New Approach to Explaining Sick Role Behavior in Low Income Populations." *American Journal of Public Health* 64 (1974): 205-216.

Belloc, N. B. "Relationship of Health Practices and Mortality" *Preventive Medicine* 2(1973): 67-81.

Boyce, Tom, and Michael, Max. "Nine Assumptions of Western Medicine." *Man and Medicine* 1 (Summer 1976): 311-335.

Brody, Howard. "The Systems View of Man: Implications for Medicine, Science and Ethics." *Perspectives in Biology and Medicine* 17 (1973): 71-92.

Cohen, Raquel. "Principles of Preventive Mental Health Programs for Ethnic Minority Populations." *American Journal of Psychiatry* 128 (June 1972): 79-83.

Dubos, René. "The Diseases of Civilization: Achievements and Illusions." In *Mainstreams of Medicine: Essays on the Social and Intellectual Context of Medical Practice,* Edited by Lester King. Austin: University of Texas Press, 1971.

Engel, George L. "The Need for a New Medical Model: A Challenge for Biomedicine" *Science* 196 (April 8, 1977): 129-36.

Freyman, John G. "Medicine's Great Schism: Prevention vs. Care." *Medical Care* 20, 7 (July 1975): 533.

Glazier, William H. "The Task of Medicine." *Scientific American* 228 (April 1973): 13-17.

Hayes-Bautista, David, and Harveston, Dominic S. "Holistic Health Care." *Social Policy* 7 (March/April 1977): 7-13.

Hilleboe, Herman E. "Preventing Future Shock: Health Developments in the 1960's and Imperative for the 1970's." *American Journal of Public Health,* February 1972, p. 139.

Parsons, Talcott. "Illness and the Role of the Physician: A Sociological Perspective." In *Medical Care: Readings in the Sociology of Medical Institutions,* Edited by W. Richard Scott and Edmund H. Volkort. New York: Wiley, 1966.

Rosenstock, Irwin M. "Why People Use Health Services." *Millbank Memorial Fund Quarterly* 44 (July 1966): 94-127.

Russell, Robert D. "Teaching for Meaning in Health Education: The Concept Approach." *Journal of School Health* (January 1966): 13-14.

Sheldon, Alan. "Toward a General Theory of Disease and Medical Care." In *Systems and Medical Care,* Edited by Alan Sheldon, Frank Baker, and Curtis P. McLaughlin. Cambridge: MIT Press, 1970.

Spark, Richard. "The Case Against Regular Physicals." *New York Times Magazine* 25 July, 1976, pp. 10, 11, 38-41.

Spector, Manuel, and Spector, Rachel E. "Is Prevention Myth or Reality?" *Health Education* 8 (July-August 1977): 23-25.

Suchman, Edward A. "Stages of Illness and Medical Care." *Journal of Health and Human Behavior* 6 (Fall 1965): 114-28.

CHAPTER 3

Familial Folk Remedies

"As modern medicine becomes more impersonal, people are recalling with some wistfulness old country cures administered by parents and grandparents over the generations."[1] If this practice occurs within the general population, does it not also occur among those who deliver health care? Given the problem that was described in the first two chapters—that is, the difficulty of defining health and illness—it can be assumed that the reader may also have little or no working knowledge of personally practiced "folk medicine" within his own family. In addition to exploring the already described questions regarding the definitions of health and illness, readers should describe how they treat their own minor illnesses and how they prevent illness. A common form of self-medication and treatment tends to be the use of aspirin for headaches and colds, or occasionally taking diet supplements with vitamins. Initially, one may admit to using tea, honey, and lemon, and hot or cold compresses for headaches and/or minor aches and pains. For the most part, however, our answers tend to be more oriented toward the health-care system for the treatment of minor illness. In an attempt to bring to consciousness one's knowledge of familial folk remedies, the following procedure is useful.

Interviewing your maternal* grandmother or grandaunt, and/or your mother, obtain answers to the following questions:

1. What is the family's ethnic background?
   Country of origin?
   Religion?
2. What did *they* do to maintain health?
   What did *their mothers* do?
3. What did *they* do to prevent illness?
   What did *their mothers* do?
4. What home remedies did *they* use to treat illness?
   What did *their mothers* use?

There are multiple reasons for structuring this exploration around your own familial past. First, it draws your attention to your own ethnic heritage and belief system. Many of your personal daily habits relate to early socialization practices that are passed on by parents or additional significant others. Many behaviors are both unconscious and habitual, and much of what you believe and practice is passed on in this manner. By digging into the past, remote and recent, you can recall some of the rituals you observed either your parents or grandparents perform: you are then better able to realize their origin and significance. There are many beliefs and practices that are similar across ethnic groups. Socialization patterns also tend to be similar among ethnic groups. Religion also plays a role in the perception of, interpretation of, and behavior in health and illness.

The maternal side is selected for the interview because in today's society of interethnic and interreligious marriages, it is assumed that the ethnic beliefs and practices related to health and illness of the family will be more in tune with the mother's family than with the father's. By and large, nurturance has been the domain of women in most cultures and societies. The mother tends to be the individual within a family who cares for family members when illness occurs; she also tends to be the prime mover in preventing illness and seeking health care. It is the mother who tells the child what and how much to eat and drink, when to go to bed, and how to dress in inclement weather. She

---

*An explanation for this choice follows in the text.

shares her knowledge and experience with her offspring, but usually the daughter is singled out for such experiential sharing.

A second reason for this examination of familial health practices is to sensitize yourself to the role that your own ethnic heritage has played in personal beliefs and practices with regard to health and illness. You must again reanalyze the concepts of health and illness with this idea in mind and, once again, view your own definitions from another perspective. If the familial background is presented in a class setting, the peer group can see these individuals in a different light: a group observes similarities and differences among its members in health and illness perspectives. You discover peer beliefs and practices that you originally had no idea existed. You may then be able to identify the "why" behind many daily health habits, practices, and beliefs.

Quite often you may be amazed to discover the origins of these health practices. Reflecting on the origin of health-practice habits may also help to explain the "mysterious" behavior of a roommate or friend. It is interesting to discover crossethnic practices within one's own group. There are always people who believed that a given practice was an "original," practiced only by their family. Many religious customs, such as "the blessing of the throats," are now conceptualized in terms of health and illness behavior. Table 2 lists a sample of responses to the questions that students obtained from members of the maternal side of their families.

"CONSCIOUSNESS-RAISING"

Recognizing Similarities

In my experience, as the group discussion continues people realize that many personal beliefs and practices do in fact differ from what they are being taught in nursing education to accept as the "right" way of doing things. Participants begin to admit that they do not seek medical care when the first symptoms of illness appear; on the contrary, one usually delays seeking care and often elects to self-treat at home. One also recognizes that there are a multitude of primary preventive and health-maintenance acts

Table 2. Family Health Histories Obtained from Students

Ethnic Background and Religion	Health Maintenance
Black and Indian (Native American), Baptist	Eat balanced meals three times a day. Dress right for the weather
Black African (Ethiopia), Orthodox Christian	Keep the area clean. Pray every morning when getting up from bed.
English, Episcopal	Thorough diet, vitamins. Enough sleep. Cod liver oil.
English, Baptist	Eat well; daily walks; read; keep warm
English, Catholic	Lots of exercise; proper sleep; lots of walking; no drinking or smoking; hard work. Bedroom window open at night. Take baths. Never dirty clothing. Good housekeeping. Immediate clean-up after meals; wash pans before meals. Rest.

Prevention	Home Treatment
Keep everything clean and sterile. Stay away from people who are sick. Regular checkups. Blackstrap molasses.	*Bloody nose:* Place keys on a chain around neck to stop. *Sore throat:* Suck yolks out of egg shell; honey and lemon; baking soda, salt, warm water, onions around the neck; salt water to gargle.
Eat hot food, such as pepper, fresh garlic, lemon.	Eat hot and sour foods, such as lemons, fresh garlic, hot mustard, red pepper. Make a kind of medicine from leaves and roots of plants mixed together. *Colds:* Hot boiled milk with honey. *Evil eye:* They put some kind of plant root on fire and make the man who has the evil eye smile and the man talks about his illness.
	Colds and sore throats: Camphor on chest and red scarves around chest
	Earache: Honey and tea, warm cod liver oil in ear; stay in bed *Cold:* Heat up glass and put on back
Maintain a good diet; fresh vegetables; vitamins; little meat; lots of fish; no fried foods; lots of sleep. Strict enforcement of life-style. Keep kitchen at 90°F in winter and house will be warm.	*Cuts:* Wet tobacco *Colds:* Chicken soup; herb tea made from roots; alcohol concoctions; Vicks and hot towels on chest; lots of fluids, rest; Vicks, sulfur, and molasses *Sore Throat:* Four onions and sugar steeped to heal and soothe the throat *Rashes:* Burned linen and cornstarch

Table 2. *(Continued)*

Ethnic Background and Religion	Health Maintenance
French (France), Catholic	Proper food; rest; proper clothing; cod liver oil daily
French Canadian, Catholic	Wear rubbers in the rain and dress warmly; take part in sports; active body; lots of sleep
Nova Scotian, Catholic	Sleep; proper foods

Prevention	Home Treatment
Every spring give sulfur and molasses for three days as a laxative to get rid of worms.	*Colds:* Rub chest with Vicks; honey
Sulfur and molasses in the spring to clear the system. Cod liver oil in orange juice. No "junk foods;" play outside; walk; daily use of Geritol; camphor on clothes; balanced meals	*Colds:* Brandy with warm milk; honey and lemon juice; hot poultice on the chest; tea, whiskey, and lemon *Back pain:* Mustard packs *Rashes:* Oatmeal baths *Sore throat:* Wrap raw potatoes in sack and tie around neck; soap and water enemas *Warts:* Rub potato on wart, run outside and throw it over left shoulder
Cut up some onions and put them on back of stove to cook; feed them to all	*Colds:* Boil carrots until jellied, add honey; as expectorant boil onions, add honey *Sore throat:* Coat a tablespoon of molasses with black pepper *Earache:* Put few drops of heated camphorated oil in ear; melted chicken fat and sugar, put in ear *Psoriasis:* Hang a piece of lead around the neck *Earache with infection:* To drain the infection, cut a piece of salt pork about 2 inches long and 3/4-inch thick and insert it into the infected ear and leave for a few days *Cold in the back:* Alcohol was put in a small metal container, a piece of cotton on a stick was placed in the alcohol, ignited, and put in a *banky* (a type of glass resembling a whisky

Table 2. *(Continued)*

Ethnic Background and Religion	Health Maintenance
Nova Scotian, Catholic (Continued)	
Canadian, Catholic	Cleanliness Food: people should eat well (fat people used to be considered healthy) Prayer: health was always mentioned in prayer
German (United States), Catholic	Wear rubbers; never go barefoot; long underwear and stockings. Wash before meals; change clothes often. Take shots. Take aspirin.

Prevention	Home Treatment
	glass); this was put on the back where the cold was and left for half an hour and a hickylike rash would develop; it was believed that the rash would drain the cold *Skin ulcer and infection:* A sharp blade was sterilized and used to make a small incision in the skin, and live blood suckers were placed in the opening; they would drain the infection out; when the blood sucker was full, it would fall to a piece of paper, be bled, placed in alcohol, and reused
Sleep. Lots of good food. Elixirs containing herbs and brewed, given as a vitamin tonic Wear camphor around the neck to ward off any evil spirit; use Father John's medicine November to May	*Kidney problems:* Herbal teas *Colds:* Hot lemons *Infected wounds:* Raw onions placed on wounds *Cough:* Shot of whiskey *Sinuses:* Camphor placed in a pouch and pinned to the shirt *Fever:* Lots of blankets and heat make you sweat out a fever *Headache:* Lie down and rest in complete darkness *Aches and pains:* Hot epsom salt baths *Eye infections:* Potatoes are rubbed on them or a gold wedding ring is placed on them and the sign of the cross is made three times
No sweets at meals. Drink glass of water at meals. Cod liver oil. Plenty of milk. Exercise. Spring tonic: sulfured molasses.	*Coughs:* Honey and vinegar *Earache:* Few drops of warm milk in the ear; laxatives when needed *Swollen glands or mumps:* Put pepper on salt pork and tie around the neck

Table 2. *(Continued)*

Ethnic Background and Religion	Health Maintenance
German (United States), Catholic (Continued)	Good diet.
Irish (United States), Catholic	Good food, balanced diet. Vitamins. "Blessing of the throat." Wear holy medals, green scapular. Dress warmly. Plenty of rest. Avoid "fast foods." Attitudes were important: "Good living habits and good thinking;" "Eat breakfast — if late for school, eat a good breakfast and be a little later;" "Don't be afraid to spend on groceries — you won't spend on the doctor later." Keep clean Keep feet warm and dry Outdoor exercise, enjoy fresh air and sunshine.

Prevention	Home Treatment
	Constipation: Ivory soap suppositories
	Sore throat: Saltwater gargle
	Sore back: Hot mustard plaster
	Sty: Cold tea leaf compress
	Cramps: Ginger tea
	Coughs: Honey and lemon; hot water and Vicks; boiled onion water, honey, and lemon
	Fever: Mix whiskey, water, and lemon juice and drink before bed; causes person to perspire and break fever
	Headache: Boil a beef bone and break up toast in the broth and drink
	Recovery diet: Boil milk and shredded wheat and add a dropped egg—first thing eaten after an illness
Clean out bowels with senna for eight days	See doctor only in emergency
Every spring, drink a mixture of sulfur and molasses to clean blood.	*Fever:* Spirits of niter on a dry sugar cube or mix with water; cold baths; alcohol rubdowns
Avoid sick people.	*Earache:* Heat salt, put in stocking behind the ear
Onions under the bed to keep nasal passages clear.	*Colds:* Tea and toast; chest rub; vaporizer; hot lemonade and a tablespoon of whiskey; mustard plasters; Vicks Vaporub on chest; whiskey; Vicks in nostrils; hot milk with butter, soups, honey, hot toddies, lemon juice, and egg whites; Ipecac ("cruel but good medicine"); whiskey with hot water and sugar; soak feet in hot water and sip hot lemonade
During flue season, tie a bag of camphor around the neck.	
Never go to bed with wet hair.	
Eat lots of oily foods.	
Take Father John's Medicine every so often.	
Prevent evil spirits: Don't look in mirror at night and close closet doors.	
Drink senna tea at every vacation; cleans out the system.	*Coughs:* Cough syrup (available on

Table 2. *(Continued)*

Ethnic Background and Religion	Health Maintenance
Irish (United States), Catholic (Continued)	Brush teeth, if out of toothpaste use table salt, or ivory soap, or Dr. Lyon's Tooth Powder. Be clean, wear clean clothes. Early to bed ("Rest is the best medicine.")

Prevention	Home Treatment
Maintain a strong family with lots of love. Be goal-oriented. Nurture a strong religious faith.	stove all winter) made from honey and whiskey; Vicks on chest; mustard plaster on chest; onion-syrup cough medicine; steam treatment; swallow Vicks; linseed poultice on chest; mustard plaster on chest; flaxseed poultice on back, red flannel cloth soaked in hot water and placed on chest all night *Menstrual cramps:* Hot milk sprinkled with ginger; shot of whiskey, glass of warm wine; warm teas; hot-water bottle on stomach *Splinters:* Flax seed poultice *Sunburn:* Apply vinegar; put milk on cloth and apply to burn; a cold, wet tea bag on small areas such as eyelids *Nausea and other stomach ailments:* Hot teas; castor oil; hot ginger ale; bay leaf; cup of hot boiled water; potato for upset stomach; baking soda; gruel *Sore throat:* Paint throat with iodine, honey and lemon, Karo syrup; paint with kerosene oil internally with a rag and then tie a sock around the neck; paint with iodine or mercurochrome and gargle with salt and water, honey, melted Vicks *Insect bites:* Vasoline or boric acid *Boils:* Oatmeal poultice *Cuts:* Boric acid *Headaches:* Hot poultice on forehead; hot facecloth; cold, damp cloth to forehead; in general, stay in bed, get plenty of rest and sleep, a glass

Table 2. *(Continued)*

Ethnic Background and Religion	Health Maintenance
Irish (United States), Catholic (Continued)	
Iran (United States), Islam	Cleanliness. Diet.
Italian (Italy), Catholic	Hearty and varied nutritional intake; lots of fruit, pasta, wine (even for children), cheese, homegrown vegetables, and salads; exercise in form of physical labor; molasses on a piece of bread or oil and sugar on bread; hard bread (good for the teeth). Pregnancy: Two weeks early: girl Two weeks late: boy Heartburn: baby with lots of hair Eat (solved emotional and physical problems); fruit at end of meal cleans teeth; early to bed and early to rise

Prevention	Home Treatment
	of juice about once an hour, aspirin, and lots of food to get back strength *Styes:* Hot tea bag to area
Dress properly for the season and weather; keep feet from getting wet in the rain. Inoculations	*Sore throat:* Gargle with vinegar and water *Cough:* Honey and lemon *Indigestion:* Baking soda and water *Sore muscles:* Alcohol and water *Rashes:* Apply corn starch
Garlic cloves strung on a piece of string around the neck of infants and children to prevent colds and "evil" stares from other people, which they believed could cause headaches and a pain or stiffness in the back or neck (a piece of red ribbon or cloth on an infant served the same purpose). Keep warm in cold weather. Keep feet warm. Eat properly. Never wash hair or bathe during period. Never wash hair before going outdoors or at night. Stay out of drafts. To prevent "evil" in the newborn a scissor was kept open under the mattress of the crib To prevent bowlegs and keep ankles straight, up to the age of 6-8 months a bandage was wrapped around the baby from the waist to the feet	Chicken soup for everything from colds to having a baby *Boils:* Cooked oatmeal wrapped in a cloth (steaming hot) applied to drain pus *Headache:* Fill a soup bowl with cold water and put some olive oil in a large spoon; hold the spoon over the bowl in front of the person with the headache; while doing this, recite words in Italian and place index finger in the oil in the spoon; three drops of oil drop from the finger into the bowl; by the diameter of the circle the oil makes when it spreads in the water the severity of the headache can be determined (larger = more severe); after this is done three times the headache is gone. Kerchief with ice in it is wrapped around the head; mint tea. *Upset stomach:* Herb tea made with herbs sent from Italy *Sore throat:* Honey; apply Vicks on

Table 2. *(Continued)*

Ethnic Background and Religion	Health Maintenance
Italian (Italy), Catholic (Continued)	

Prevention	Home Treatments
If infants got their nights and days mixed up, they were tied upside down and turned all the way around	throat at bedtime and wrap up the throat *Sprains:* Beat egg whites, apply to part, wrap part up *Fever:* Cover with blankets to sweat it out *Cramps:* Creme de menthe *Poison ivy:* Yellow soap suds *Colic:* Warm oil on stomach *Acne:* Apply baby's urine *Sucking thumb:* Apply hot pepper to thumb *High blood pressure:* In Italy for high blood pressure, colonies of blood suckers were kept in clay, where they were born; the person with high blood pressure would have a blood sucker put on his fanny, where it would suck blood; it was thought that this would lower his blood pressure; the blood suckers would then be thrown in ashes and would then throw up the blood they had sucked from the person. If the blood sucker died, it alerted the person to see a doctor because it sometimes meant that there was something wrong with the person's blood *Stomach ache:* Carnilla and maloa (herbs) added to boiled water *Colds:* Boiled wines; coffee with anisette *Pimples:* To draw contents, apply hot flaxseed *Toothache:* Whiskey applied topically

Table 2. *(Continued)*

Ethnic Background and Religion	Health Maintenance
Italian (Italy), Catholic (Continued)	
Norwegian (Norway), Lutheran	Cod liver oil. Cleanliness. Rest.
Polish (United States), Catholic	Use of physician Eating good, nutritious foods Plenty of rest Cod liver oil
Swedish (United States), Protestant	Eat well-balanced meals. A lot of walking. Routine medical exams. Cod liver oil.

Prevention	Home Treatment
	Backache: Apply hot oatmeal in a sock; place a silver dollar on the sore area, light a match to it; while the match is burning put a glass over the silver dollar and then slightly lift the glass, and this causes a suction, which is said to lift the pain out
	To build up blood: Eggnog with brandy; Marsala wine and milk
	Muscle pain: Heat up carbon leaves (herb) and bundle in a hot cloth to make a pack (soothes any discomfort)
Immunizations	*Colds and sore throat:* Hot peppermint drink and Vicks Vaporub.
Exercise; good diet; eat fresh, home-grown foods; work; good personal hygiene	*Headache:* Take aspirin, hot liquids
	Sore muscles: Heating pads and hot compresses
	Colds: Drink hot liquids, chicken soup, honey
Eat an apple a day	*Cough:* Warm milk and butter
"I don't do a blooming thing;" eat well	*Run down and tired:* Eat a whole head of lettuce
Eat sorghum molasses for general all-round good health	*Sick:* Lots of juices and decarbonated ginger ale; lots of rest
Dress appropriately for weather	*Upset stomach:* Baking soda
Blessing of the throats on St. Blaise Day	*Sore throat:* Gargle with salt and take honey in milk; herringbone wrapped in flannel around the neck
	Anemia: Cod liver oil
	Bee stings: Poultice

Table 2. *(Continued)*

Ethnic Background and Religion	Health Maintenance
Swedish (United States), Protestant (Continued)	
Eastern Europe (United States), Jewish	Go to doctor when sick (mother). Health care for others, not self (mother). Reluctantly sought medical help (grandmother). Health for self not a priority (grandmother). Physician twice a year (mother). Doctor only when pregnant (grandmother).
Austrian (United States), Jewish	Eat wholesome foods, homegrown fruits and vegetables. Bake own bread

that we have learned in school but choose not to comply with! Sometimes one discovers that she or he is following an entire regimen for a multitude of health-related problems, and does not seek any outside intervention.

Another facet of such a discussion is that it exposes participants to the similarities that exist among them in terms of prevention and health maintenance. To their surprise and delight, many of

Prevention	Home Treatment
	Lumbago: Drink a yeast mixture *Black eye:* Leeches *Earache:* Warm oil *Congestion:* Steamy bathroom *Fever:* Blankets to sweat it out
Observe precautions, such as dressing warmly, not going out with wet hair; getting enough rest, staying in bed if not feeling well (mother). Not much to prevent illness—very ill today with chronic diseases (grandmother) Vitamins and water pills	*Colds:* Fluids, aspirin, rest *Stomach upset:* Eat light and bland foods *Muscle aches:* Massage with alcohol *Sore throat:* Gargle with salt water; tea with lemon and honey *Insomnia:* Glass of wine Chicken soup used by mother and grandmother
Camphor around the neck (in the winter) in a small cloth bag to prevent measles and scarlet fever	*Sore throat:* Go to the village store, find a salted herring, wrap it in a towel, put it around the neck, and let it stay there overnight; gargle with salt water *Boils:* Fry chopped onions, make a compress and apply to the infections

their daily acts that are taken for granted directly relate to methods of maintaining health and preventing illness.

As is common in most large groups, students seem to be shy at the beginning of this exploration. However, as more and more individual members of the group are willing to share their experiences, other students feel more comfortable and share more readily. A classroom tactic I have used to break the ice is to reveal an experience I had upon the birth of my first child. My mother-in-law, a woman from Eastern Europe, drew a circle around the child's crib with her fingers and spat on the baby three times to prevent the evil spirits from harming him. Once such an anecdote is shared, other participants have less difficulty in remembering similar events that may have taken place in their own homes!

Students have a wide variety of feelings about the self-care practices of their families. One feeling discussed by many students is *shame*. A number of students express a dichotomy in their attitudes: they cannot decide whether to believe these old ways or to drop them and adopt the more modern ones they are learning in nursing school. (This is an example of cognitive dissonance.) Many admit that this is the first time they have disclosed these beliefs and practices in public, and they are relieved and amazed to discover similarity among other peoples. The acts may have different names or be performed in a slightly different manner, but the uniting thread among them is to prevent evil (illness) and to maintain good (health)!

Transference to Clients

The effects of such a verbal catharsis are long remembered and often quoted and/or referred to throughout the remainder of a course. The awareness that we gain helps us to better understand the behavior and beliefs of our patients. Given this understanding, we are comfortable enough to ask patients how they interpret a symptom and how they think it ought to be treated. Thus we begin to be more sensitive to people who, for one reason or another, delay in seeking health care or fail to comply with preventive measures and treatment regimens. We come to recognize that we do the same thing. I believe that the increased familiarity with home health practices and remedies helps us to project this awareness—and understanding—to the clients who are served.

When analyzed from a "scientific" perspective, the majority of these practices do have a sound basis. In the area of health maintenance (Table 2) one notes an almost universal adherence to activities that include rest, balanced diet, and exercise.

In the area of prevention there are various differences—ranging from visiting a physician to wearing a clove of garlic around the neck. While the purpose of wearing garlic around the neck is "to keep the evil spirit away," the act also forces people to stay away: what better way to cut down exposure to wintertime colds than to avoid close contact with people?!

One person remembered that during her childhood her mother forced her to wear garlic around her neck. Like most children, she did not like to be different from the rest of her schoolmates. As time went on, she began to have frequent colds, and her mother could not understand why this was happening. The mother followed her child to school some weeks later and discovered that she removed the garlic on her way to school—hiding it under a rock and then replacing it on the way home. There was quite a battle between the mother and daughter! The youngster did not like this method of prevention because her peers mocked her.

A discussion of home remedies is of further interest when each of the methods presented is analyzed for its possible "medical" analogy and also for its prevalence among ethnic groups. Many of these practices, to the surprise and relief of students, tend to run throughout ethnic groups but have different names or contain different ingredients.

In this day of computers and sophisticated medicine with transplants and intricate surgery, the most prevalent need expressed by people who practice folk medicine is to remove the "evil" that may be the cause of the health problem. As students we analyze and discuss a given problem and its folk treatments and we begin to see how "evil" continues to be considered the cause of illness and how often the treatment is then designed to remove it.

Each person testifies to the efficacy of a given remedy. Many state that when their grandmothers and/or mothers shared these remedies with them, they experienced great feelings of nostalgia for the good old days when things seemed so simple. Some people may express a desire to return to these practices of yesteryear, whereas others openly confess that they continue to use such measures even now—sometimes in addition to what a physician tells them to use or often without even bothering to consult a physician.

The goal of this kind of consciousness-raising session is to reawaken the participant to the types of health practices within her own family. The other purpose of the sharing is to make known the similarities and differences that exist as part of a crossethnic phenomenon. At this point, a great deal of myth-debunking occurs. We are intrigued to discover the wide range of beliefs that exist among our peers' families. We had assumed that these people thought and believed the same as we did. For the first time, we individually and collectively realize that we *all* practice a certain amount of folk medicine, that we *all* have ethnically specific ways of treating illness, and that we, too, often delay in seeking professional health care. We learn that most people prefer to treat themselves at home, and that they have their own ways of treating a particular set of symptoms—with or without a pre-scribed medical regimen. The previously held notion that "every-body does it this way" is shattered.

REFERENCE

1. Frances Kennett. *Folk Medicine—Fact and Fiction: Age-Old Cures, Alternative Medicine, Natural Remedies* (New York: Crescent Books, 1976), p. 9.

UNIT II
Issues of Delivery and Acceptance of Health Care

This unit covers the broad topics that relate to the acquisition and utilization of health-care sources. The overall theme encompasses the problems that the client encounters.

Chapter 4 explores the health-care delivery system on the experiential level, rather than attempting to recite a synopsis of health-care delivery. Enlarging upon a theme introduced earlier, Chapter 5 explores culture and ethnicity—analyzing the impact that ethnic background may have on perception of health and illness. Chapter 6 discusses "healing"—both ancient and modern, with a number of illustrative examples.

Unit 2 should enable the reader to:

1. Understand the universal problems encountered in the utilization of the health-care system;

2. Understand how organized medical practice serves as an institution of social control;
3. Identify the various types of people who practice the "art" of healing.

CHAPTER 4
The Delivery of Health Care

Before you begin to read this chapter, please deal with the following issues:

1. Who is the first person you turn to when you are ill?
2. Who do you go to and where do you go to from there?
3. You have just moved to a new location. You do not know a single person in this community. How do you find health-care resources?
4. Call the county medical society in your area and request the name of a surgeon. Now make an appointment with this doctor. (Assume you have a health problem that requires surgery.)
5. Visit an emergency room in a large municipal hospital. Visit an emergency room in a small community hospital. Spend several hours quietly observing what occurs in each setting.
   a. How long do patients wait to be seen?
   b. Are patients called by name?
   c. Are relatives or friends allowed into the treatment room with the patient?

American medicine, the pride of the nation for many years, stands on the brink of chaos. To be sure, our medical practitioners have their great moments of drama and triumph. But, much of U.S. medical care, particularly the everyday business of preventing and treating illness, is inferior in quality, wastefully dispensed, and inequitably financed. Medical manpower and facilities are so maldistributed that large segments of the population, especially the urban poor and those in rural areas, get virtually no care at all, even though their illnesses are most numerous and, in a medical sense, often easy to cure.[1]

—John Knowles

The timeliness of this quotation is easily demonstrated with a presentation of current data. Although there are some people today who maintain that, in fact, the health of the nation is no longer in crisis, one need only reflect on the material that follows* to conclude that Dr. Knowles' observations are still accurate.

1. Health resources for the Latino *barrio* (community) in Detroit are nonsystemic, haphazard, and of an an acute or episodic nature. The underemployed or unemployed worker has little or no access to comprehensive health care. For these workers, a routine visit to a clinic can result in severe financial strain.[2]

2. Hispanic males aged 15 to 45 have horrifyingly high death rates compared with their contemporaries of other backgrounds. The infant mortality rate continues to be relatively higher among the Puerto Ricans in New York compared with the general population. It is reported that the "children from 6 to 11 who are from families with incomes under $3,000 per year average 3.5 dental caries per year; however, children from families (other than Hispanic) with incomes over $15,000 per year average less than one carie per year."[3]

3. Three-fourths of the nation's retarded children are found in impoverished rural and urban slums. A child from a low-income family is 15 times more

*These data were presented at the American Public Health Association's Annual Meeting (Chicago) in November 1975.

likely to be diagnosed as retarded than a child from a high-income family.[4]

4. A study in Santa Clara County, California, pointed out that, for the Latino population, motor-vehicle traffic accidents ranked as the fourth leading cause of death; cirrhosis of the liver was fifth; and diabetes was sixth. For the white population, traffic accidents and cirrhosis of the liver ranked eighth and ninth; diabetes did not even appear among the ten leading causes of death. In addition, deaths among Latino infants are nearly three times that of the white population.[5]

5. In San Antonio, Texas, inadequate health insurance coverage for Chicano workers continues to be a major problem.[6]

I believe that these examples graphically illustrate the words of Dr. Knowles. However, as mentioned, there are those who contend that the crises of health-care delivery and increasing costs that were feared in the early 1970s no longer exist. Dr. David E. Rogers and Dr. Robert J. Blendon recently stated: "Things within the health care system have gotten better." They cite the following data[7] to support their claims.

1. Today, physician care is less difficult to obtain than it was five years ago; between 1969 and 1975, personal-physician visits rose by 20 percent.

2. There are indications that medical care is more available to the poor and to Blacks; the pattern has changed since 1965 to 1975, with the poor seeing physicians slightly more often than people of high income.*

3. Death rates have been falling for the last seven years.

4. Infant mortality rates have declined to 16.1 per 1000 live births in 1975 from 26 per 1000 live births in 1960.

*Rogers and Blendon fail to mention the quality of care, the reason for seeking care, or the percentage of the Black population that is included in this formulation.

Rogers and Blendon conclude their article with this statement: "These broad changes do not suggest an overall worsening in the health situation for those who live in the United States. We must be doing some things right, and there seems room for some cautious optimism about the future."[7]

COMMON PROBLEMS IN HEALTH-CARE DELIVERY

On the one hand, it is refreshing to read a report such as the one cited above. However, if we carefully examine the background information as well as the counter arguments, we are likely to be less optimistic than Rogers and Blendon would like us to be. There are innumerable problems within the health-care delivery system today. There are problems that affect all of us, and there are those that are specific to the poor and to minority populations. Statistics alone cannot obfuscate these issues. Changes in death rates and infant mortality rates do not change morbidity rates. To say that people are utilizing more physicians in no way indicates that they are necessarily receiving quality care. If the frequency of going to a physician has increased, it may signify more illness rather than more use in general. It may mean that physicians are not treating patients properly, so that people must keep returning until the right combinations of treatments are found, presented, and followed.

It has been suggested that the health-care delivery system fosters and maintains a childlike dependence and depersonalized condition for the consumer. The following section describes problems experienced by most consumers of health care.

Consumer Experiences

"Finding Where the Appropriate Care Is Offered at a Reasonable Price"[8]

The following example demonstrates how difficult it is for even a knowledgeable consumer to receive adequate care. In the summer of 1976, I was on vacation with my 11-year-old daughter. She complained of a sore throat for two days and, when she did not improve on the third day, I decided to take her to a pediatrician and have a throat culture taken. She was running a low-grade fever, and I suspected a strep throat. I phoned the emergency room of a local teaching hospital for the name of a pediatrician, but I was instructed to "bring her in." I questioned the practicality of using an emergency room but the friendly voice on the other end of the line assured me: "If you have health insurance and the child has a sore throat, this is the best place to come." After a rather long wait, we were seen by an intern who was beginning his first day in pediatrics. To my dismay and chagrin, the young man appeared to have no idea of how to proceed. The resident entered and patiently demonstrated to the fledgling intern—using my daughter—how to go about doing a physical examination on a child. Since I had brought the child to the emergency room merely for a throat culture, I felt that what they were doing was unnecessary and said so. After much delay, the throat culture was taken; we were told we could leave, and to call back in 48 hours for the report. As we left the cubicle, we had to pass another cubicle with an open curtain—where a woman was vomiting all over herself, the bed, and the equipment while another intern was attempting to pass a gastric tube. Needless to say, my daughter was distressed by the sight which she could not help but witness. The reward for this trial was a bill for $70. The hospital charged $25 for the use of the emergency room and $45 for the throat culture. I expressed shock and outrage at such an inflated bill.

Two days later I called back for the report. It could not be located. When it was finally "found," the result was negative. I took issue with this because it took 30 minutes for them to find the report. Perhaps this sounds a bit overstated; however, I had the feeling that they told me it was negative just to get me off the phone.

I have related this actual experience to bring out two major points. First, it is not easy to obtain what I, as a health-care provider, would consider to be a rather minor procedure. Second—and more important to those who may be down-and-out financially—it is expensive!

The average person who undergoes such an experience may very well have no idea of what is really going on in the surrounding environment. When health care is sought, one should have access to professionally given examinations and treatment. When one is seeking the results of a laboratory test, the results should be immediately available at the agreed-upon time and place instead of being lost in a jungle of bureaucracy.

"Finding One's Way Amidst the Many Available Types of Medical Care"[9]

A story illustrating this phenomenon in a broad context is that of a friend who experienced minor gastric problems from time to time. She initially sought help from a family physician. He was unable to treat the problem adequately; therefore, she decided to go elsewhere. However, for many reasons—including anger, embarrassment, and fear of reprisal—she chose not to tell the family physician that she was dissatisfied with his care and to request a referral. She was, for all intents and purposes, on her own in terms of securing an appointment with either a gastroenterologist or a surgeon. She very quickly discovered that no physician who was a specialist in gastroenterology would see her on a self-referral. In order to get an appointment, she had to ask her own general practitioner for a referral or else seek initial help from another general practitioner or internist. Since she had little money to spend on a variety of physicians, she decided to wait to see what would happen. In this instance, happily, she has been fortunate: she has had few further problems.

However, numerous people experience the problem of seeking a second opinion or trying to locate a new physician if they are dissatisfied with their current one. Most individuals, unlike my friend, are not lucky enough to have their problems resolve themselves and must go in search of additional medical advice.

As a teaching and learning experience, I ask students to describe how they go about selecting a physician and where they go for health care. The younger students in the class generally utilize the services of their families' physicians. The older and/or married students often have doctors other than those with whom they "grew up." These latter students are generally quite willing to share the trials and tribulations that they have experienced. When given the freedom to express their actions and reactions, most admit to having a great deal of difficulty in getting what they perceive to be *good* health care. A number of the older students state that they select a physician on the staff of the institution where they are employed: they have had an opportunity to see him at work and can judge, first hand, whether he is "good" or "bad." One mother stated that she worked in pediatrics during her pregnancy solely to discover who was the best pediatrician. A newly married student stated that she planned to work in the delivery room to see which obstetrician delivered a baby with the greatest amount of concern for both the mother and the child.

That is all well and good for members of the nursing profession. But what about the average lay person who does not have access to this resource? This question alerts the students to the uniqueness of their personal situations and exposes them to the immensity of the problem that the average person experiences. After individual experiences are shared, the class can move on to work-through this area more completely with a case study such as that described below.

Ms. B. is a new resident in this city. She discovered a lump in her breast and does not know where to turn. How does she go about finding a doctor? Where does she go? What does she do?

One initial course of action is to call the American Cancer Society for advice. From there, she is instructed to call the County Medical Society—the American Cancer Society is not allowed to give out physicians' names. During a phone call to the County Medical Society she is given the names of three physicians in her part of the city; from there she is on her own in attempting to get an appointment with one of them. It is not unknown for a stranger to call a physician's office and to be told: (1) "The doctor is no longer seeing any additional new patients;" (2) "There is a six-month wait;" or (3) "He sees no one without a proper referral."

The woman, of course, has another choice: She can go to an emergency room or a clinic. But then she discovers that the wait in the emergency room is intolerable for her. She may rationalize that because a "lump" is not really an "emergency," she should choose another route. She may then try to secure a clinic appointment, and once again she may experience a great deal of difficulty in getting an appointment at a convenient time. She may finally get one and then discover that the wait in the clinic is unduly long—which may cause her to miss a day of work, and that will entail all sorts of explanations.

"Figuring Out What the Physician Is Doing"[10]

It is not always easy for members of the health professions to understand what is happening to them when they are ill. Alas, what must it be like for the average person who has little or no knowledge of health-care routines and practices?

Pretend that you are a lay person who has just been relieved of all your clothes and given a paper dress to put on. You are lying on a table with strange eyes peering down at you. A sheet is thrown over you, and you are given terse directions—"breathe," "cough," "don't breathe," "turn," "lift your legs." You may feel without warning a cold disk on your chest or a cold hand on your back. As the physical-examination process continues, you may feel a few taps of the ribs, see a bright light shining in your eye, feel a cold tube in your ear, and gag on a stick probing the inside of your mouth. What is going on? The jargon you hear is unfamiliar. You are being poked, pushed, prodded, peered at and into, jabbed, and you do not know why. If you are female and going for your first pelvic examination, you may have no idea what to expect. Perhaps you have heard only hushed whisperings, and your level of fear and discomfort is high. Insult is added to injury when you experience the penetration of the cold, un-yielding speculum: "What is he doing now and why?"

These hypothetical situations are typical of the more everyday physical examinations that one may routinely encounter in a clinic or private physician's office. But suppose you have a more complex problem, such as a neurologic condition, for which the diagnostic procedures may indeed be painful and complicated. Have you ever had a spinal tap? A myelogram? An angiogram? Quite often, those who deliver care have not experienced the vast number of procedures that are done in diagnostic work-ups and in treatment; they have little awareness of what the patient is think-ing, feeling, and experiencing. Similarly, because the names and the purposes of the procedures are familiar to health-care workers—don't forget, this is *their* culture, *their* bailiwick, *their* turf—they may experience a great deal of difficulty in appreciating why the patient cannot understand what is happening.

"Finding Out What Went Wrong"[11]

What did you do the last time a patient asked to read his chart? Traditionally one uttered an authoritative "tsk," turned abruptly on white-heeled shoes, and walked briskly away. Who ever heard of such nerve? A patient asking to read his chart! In recent years, a "patient's bill of rights" has evolved. One of its mandates is that the patient has the right to read his own medical record. Experience, however, demonstrates that this right is still not granted. Suppose one enters the hospital for what is deemed to be a simple medical or surgical problem. All well and good, if everything goes according to routine. However, what happens when complications develop? The more determined the patient is to discover what the problem is or why he is experiencing complications, the more he believes that the health-care providers are trying to hide something. The cycle perpetuates itself, and a tremendous schism develops between provider and consumer. Quite often, "the conspiracy of silence" tends to grow as more questions are asked. This unpleasant situation may continue until the patient is locked outside his subjective world. It is rare for a person truly to understand unforeseen complications. Nurses all too often enter into this collusion and play the role of a silent partner with the physician and the institution.

"Overcoming the Built-in Racism and Male Chauvinism of Doctors and Hospitals"[12]

Students tend to have little difficulty in describing a multitude of incidents that help this last-named problem come alive: that they are mostly women suffices, and that they are nurses adds meaning to the problem. Classroom discussion helps to identify subtle incidents of racism and to identify them as such. For example, students may realize that Black patients may be the last to receive morning or evening care, meal trays, and so forth. If this is a "normal" occurrence on a floor, it is an indictment in itself. However, such racism may take another tack. Is it an accident that the Black person is the last patient to receive routine care, or that he has consciously been made to wait? Does the fact that the Black person may have to wait longest for water or a pill demonstrate racism on a conscious level, or is it subliminal?

Nurses recognize the subtle patronization of both themselves and of female patients. Once the situation is probed and spelled-out, the students adopt a much more realistic attitude toward the insensitivity of those who choose a racist and/or chauvinistic style of giving care. Students have noted that when they are aware of what is happening, they are better able to take steps to block future occurrences. Some have written letters to me after they have begun or returned to the practice of nursing, stating that knowing the phenomenon is universal helps them to project a stronger image in their determination to work for change.

PATHWAYS TO HEALTH SERVICES

When a health problem occurs, there is an established system whereby health-care services are obtained. The family is usually the first resource. It is in the domain of the family that the person seeks validation that what he is experiencing is indeed an illness. Once the belief is validated, health care outside of the home is sought. When one is dealing with the medical system in general, help is sought from a physician in one setting or another. It may be the private office of a general practitioner, internist, or pediatrician, or it may be in a hospital emergency room or clinic.* This is known as the level of first contact, or the *entrance* into the health-care system.[13]

The second level of care, if needed, is found at the specialist's level: in clinics, private practice, or hospitals. Obstetricians, gynecologists, surgeons, neurologists, and other specialists make up a large percentage of those who practice medicine.[14]

The third level of care is delivered within the framework of the hospitals. There are various hospitals providing in-patient care and services. Care is determined by need, whether long-term

---

*It is not unusual for a family to have a multitude of physicians providing its care, with limited or no communication between the attending physicians. Countless problems and complications erupt when a physician is not aware that there are physicians other then himself caring for a given patient. Let us not forget that in rural and remote areas, comprehensive health care is difficult to obtain. For patients who are forced to utilize the clinics of a hospital, there is certainly no continuity of care because intern and resident physicians come and go each July 1.

(as in a psychiatric setting or rehabilitation institute) or short-term (as in the acute-care setting and community hospitals).[15]

An in-depth discussion of the different kinds of hospitals—voluntary or profit-making and nonprofit institutions—is more appropriate to a book dealing solely with the delivery of health care (see the annotated bibliography at the end of this book). In our present context, the issue is: What does the patient know about such settings, and what kind of care can he expect to receive?

To many students, the problems of the ward are far removed from the scope of practice that they know from nursing school and from what they ordinarily see in a work setting (unless they choose to work in a city or county hospital). Many students assume that the care they observe and deliver in a surburban or community hospital is the universal norm. This is a fundamental error in experience and understanding, which can be corrected if students are assigned first to visit the emergency room of a city hospital and then the emergency room of a surburban hospital toward comparing and contrasting the two milieus. Unless students actually visit each setting, they fail to gain an appreciation of the major differences that occur—how vastly such facilities differ in scope of treatment and regard for patients. Students typically report that in the suburban emergency room the patients are called by name, their families wait with them, and every effort is made to hasten their visit. The contrast is astounding when they talk with people in urban emergency rooms who have waited for extended periods of time, are sometimes not addressed by name, and are not allowed to have family members come with them while they are examined. The noise and confusion are also factors that confront and dismay students who are exposed to big-city emergency rooms.

MEDICINE AS AN INSTITUTION OF SOCIAL CONTROL

The people of today's death-denying, youth-oriented society have unusually high expectations for the healers of our time. We expect a cure (or if not a cure, then the prolongation of life) as the normal outcome of any given illness.(The technology of modern health care all but dominates our expectations of treatment and our primary focus is on the *curative* aspects of medicine, not on prevention.

As control over the behavior of a person has shifted from family and church to physician, "be good" has shifted to "take your medicine." The role that physicians play within society in terms of social control is ever-growing, so that there is frequent conflict between medicine and the law over definitions of accepted codes of behavior and the relative status of the two professions in governing American life.[16] The following examples serve to illustrate the "medicalization" of society.

"Through the Expansion of What in Life Is Deemed Relevant to the Good Practice of Medicine"[17]

This factor is exemplified by the change from a specific etiologic model of disease to a multicausal one. The "partners" in this new model include greater acceptance of comprehensive medicine, the use of the computer, and the practice of preventive medicine. In preventive medicine, however, the medical person must get to the lay person before the disease occurs: clients must be sought out. Because of this, forms of social control emerge in an attempt to *prevent* disease: low-cholesterol diets, avoidance of stress, stopping smoking, getting proper and adequate exercise, and so forth.

"Through the Retention of Absolute Control over Certain Technical Procedures"[18]

This step is, in essence, the right to perform surgery and the right to prescribe drugs. In the lifespan of human beings, modern medicine can often determine life or death from the time of conception to old age through genetic counseling, abortion, surgery, and technologic devices such as computers, respirators, and life-support systems. Medicine has at its command drugs that can cure or kill—from antibiotics to the chemotherapeutic agents used to combat cancer. There are drugs to cause sleep or wakefulness, to increase or decrease the appetite, to increase or decrease levels of energy. There are drugs to relieve depression and stimulate interest. (In the United States these mood-altering drugs are consumed at a rate higher than those medications prescribed and used to treat specific diseases). In addition, medicine can control what medications are available for legal consumption.

The controversy over Laetrile is an example of how the medical establishment is thwarting the popular consumption of a drug. In spite of the "scientific" evidence that this drug is worthless, there is no evidence to date that it is harmful, and there are a significant number of people who desire to utilize it in the prevention and treatment of cancer. The ongoing battle between the proponents and opponents of Laetrile is a facinating study in the power of modern medical social control and the factions that are attacking this power. As of 1977, the proponents have made headway in lobbying for legalization of the drug in a number of states, and a Federal judicial ruling has permitted its use in individual cases.*

"Through the Retention of Near Absolute Access to Certain 'Taboo' Areas" [19]

Medicine has almost exclusive license to examine and treat that most personal of individual possessions: the mechanics of mind and body. It if can be determined that some given factor affects the body and/or the mind, then that element can be interpreted as a medical problem; it falls into the hands of medicine for treatment. Such situations currently include the normal processes of pregnancy and aging, as well as the human behavior problems of drug addiction and alcoholism.

"Through the Expansion of What in Medicine Is Deemed Relevent to the Good Practice of Life" [20]

This expansion is illustrated by the use of medical jargon to describe a state of being—such as the "health" of the nation or

---

*In July of 1977, Laetrile was the focus of much attention. Since August 1977, more studies have been conducted seeking to prove its danger. On the other hand, Laetrile has been accepted by a number of additional states. Since this remains an ongoing issue, the reader should be aware that nothing has been settled as of the time these comments were written and that the situation may change at any time.

the "health" of the economy. Any political or economic proposal or objective that enhances the "health" of those concerned wins approval.

There are numerous areas in which medicine, religion, and law overlap. One example is how, in public-health practice, law and medicine overlap in the creation of laws that establish quarantine and the need for immunization. As another example, a child is unable to enter school without proof of having received certain inoculations. They also merge in areas of sanitation, rodent control, and insect control. A legal-medical dispute can arise over the guilt or innocence of a criminal as determined by his "mental state" at the time of a crime.

There are diseases that carry a social stigma: one must be screened for tuberculosis before employment; a history of typhoid fever prevents a person from commercially handling food for life; venereal disease must be reported and treated; and even the ancient disease of leprosy continues to carry a stigma.

Abortion represents an area replete with conflict that involves law, religion, and medicine. Individuals in favor of abortion continue to believe that it is the right of the female to have an abortion and that the matter is confidential between the patient and her physician. Opponents argue on religious and moral grounds that abortion is murder. At the present time, the law sanctions abortion. In many states, however, Medicaid will no longer pay for an abortion unless the mother's life is in danger; this is making it increasingly difficult for the poor to obtain these services.

Another highly charged area of conflict involves the practice of euthanasia. With the burgeoning of technologic improvements, the definition of "death" has changed in recent years: it sometimes takes a major decision from the courts to "pull the plug," such as in the Karen Quinlan case.

Finally, one might ponder that although there are a multitude of daily practical activities that some or all of us undertake in the name of health—taking vitamins, practicing hygiene, using birth control, engaging in dietary or exercise programs—the "diseases of the rich" (cancer, heart disease, and stroke) tend to capture more public attention and funding than the diseases of the poor (malnutrition, high maternal and infant death rates, sickle cell anemia, and lead poisoning).

REFERENCES

1. John Knowles, "It's Time to Operate," *Fortune*, January 1970, p. 79.
2. Ruben G. Zamorano, "The Unemployed Detroit Latino Worker: A Health Resource Profile" (presented at the 103rd Annual Meeting of the American Public Health Association, Chicago, 16-20 November, 1975), pp. 7, 17, 19.
3. Pedro Juan Lecca et al., "Profile of Health Resources among Unemployed Puerto Ricans in the U.S." (presented at the 103rd Annual Meeting of the American Public Health Association, Chicago, 16-20 November, 1975), pp. 6, 10.
4. Ibid., p. 10.
5. Simon Dominguiz with Hector B. Garcia, "Health Resources for Unemployed Latinos in the United States." (presented at the 103rd Annual Meeting of the American Public Health Association, Chicago, 16-20 November, 1975), pp. 6-8.
6. Bernardo Eureste, "A Profile of Health Insurance Coverage for Unemployed Chicanos in San Antonio, Texas." (presented at the 103rd Annual Meeting of the American Public Health Association, Chicago, 16-20 November, 1975), p. 15.
7. David E. Rogers and Robert J. Blendon, "How Healthy Is America's Health Care?" *Boston Globe*, 10 July 1977, p. A3.
8. Barbara Ehrenreich and John Ehrenreich, *The American Health Empire: Power, Profits, and Politics* (New York: Random House, 1970), p. 4.
9. Ibid., p. 6.
10. Ibid., p. 9.
11. Ibid., p. 11.
12. Ibid., p. 12
13. John Fry, *Medicine in Three Societies* (London: Aylesbury (Bucks), MTP, 1969), p. 22.
14. Ibid.
15. Ibid., p. 23.
16. Irving Kenneth Zola, "Medicine as an Institution of Social Control," *Sociological Review* 20, no. 4, new series (November 1972): 487-504.
17. Ibid.
18. Ibid.
19. Ibid.
20. Ibid.

BIBLIOGRAPHY: THE DELIVERY OF HEALTH CARE

Bullough, Bonnie, and Bullough, Vern L. *Poverty, Ethnic Identity, and Health Care.* New York: Appleton, 1972.

This book boldly demonstrates and documents the ways in which the inadequacies of the health-care system affect the poor and members of minority groups.

Cornacchia, Harold J. *Consumer Health.* St. Louis: Mosby, 1976.

The consumer movement in the United States has made great strides in the area of protecting the public in the marketplace. The purpose of this book is to aid consumers in implementing the Bill of Rights. It describes various aspects and problems of the health-care system.

Crichton, Michael. *Five Patients.* New York: Knopf, 1970.

This interesting book explores the hospital treatment of five people. It demonstrates how hospital practice is changing in this age of technology.

Ehrenreich, Barbara, and Ehrenreich, John. *The American Health Empire: Power, Profits, and Politics.* New York: Vintage Books, 1971.

According to this team of authors, the health system is not in business for people's health. The book explores the economic aspects of health and health care and how various institutions evolve into "empires."

Freidson, Eliot. *Profession of Medicine.* New York: Dodd, Mead, 1971.

Freidson explores the word *profession.* He sees it both as an "occupation" and as an "avowal or promise." He demonstrates how the medical profession is organized, how professional performance is organized, and how illness is socially constructed.

Illich, Ivan. *Medical Nemesis: The Expropriation of Health.* London: Marion Bogars, 1975.

This excellent study deals with the topics of clinical iatrogenesis, the epidemic of modern medicine, social iatrogenesis, the medicalization of life, the destruction of medical cultures, the killing of pain, and the politics of health.

————; Zola, Irving K.; McKnight, John; Caplan, Jonathan; and Shaiken, Harley. *Disabling Professions.* Salem, N.H.: Boyars, 1977.

The authors explore the various arguments relevant to the public debate about the power of the professions. Each explores various aspects of the growing dependency of people on the professional elite who dominate, institutionalize, and ritualize all aspects of our daily lives.

Kennedy, Edward M. *In Critical Condition: The Crises in America's Health Care.* New York: Simon and Schuster, 1972.

The many problems that people often encounter when they deal with the health-care delivery system are outlined.

Millman, Marcia. *The Unkindest Cut.* New York: Morrow, 1977.

> This explosive book explores and analyzes the "back rooms" of American medicine. It examines what is done in the mortality review conferences, the emergency room, and various hospital staff meetings.

Rosenberg, Ken, and Schiff, Gordon. *The Politics of Health Care: A Bibliography.* Somerville, Mass.: New England Free Press, 1973.

> A bibliographic listing, this work cites numerous books and articles that deal with the politics of health care. It can be ordered from Health Bibliography, c/o Ken Rosenberg, 48 Aldie Street, Allston, Mass. 02134.

Silver, George. *A Spy in the House of Medicine.* Germantown, Md.: Aspen Systems, 1976.

> Why is health care so costly? How is health care delivered? What goes on in health care? These and other questions are probed in this account of health-care delivery.

FURTHER SUGGESTED READINGS

Books

Davis, Fred, editor. *The Nursing Profession: Five Sociological Essays.* New York: Wiley, 1966.

Fry, John. *Medicine in Three Societies.* London: Aylesbury (Bucks), 1969.

Fuchs, Victor R. *Who Shall Live? Health, Economics and Social Choice.* New York: Basic Books, 1974.

McKeown, Thomas. *The Role of Medicine: Dream, Mirage or Nemesis?* London: Nuffield Provincial Hospitals Trust, 1976.

Norman, John C., editor. *Medicine in the Ghetto.* New York: Appleton, 1969.

Articles

There are numerous articles available on health-care delivery; the following are a mere sampling.

Adler, Herbert M., and Hammett, V. "The Doctor-Patient Relationship Revisited: An analysis of the Placebo Effect." *Annals of Internal Medicine* 78 (1973): 595.

Fortune, January 1970.

McDermott, Walsh. "Medicine: The Public Good and One's Own." *Cornell University Medical College Alumni Quarterly* 4 (Winter 1977): 15-24.

Zola, Irving Kenneth. "Medicine as an Institution of Social Control." *Sociological Review* 20, new series (November 1972): 487-504.

CHAPTER 5
Culture, Health, and Illness

Culture is a unified whole even unto psychosis and death.

—Jules Henry, *Culture Against Man*

Health and illness can be interpreted and explained in terms of personal experience and expectations. There are many ways in which we can define our own health or illness and determine what these states mean to us in our daily lives. We learn from our own cultural and ethnic backgrounds *how* to be healthy, *how* to recognize illness, and *how* to be ill. Furthermore, the meanings attached to the notions of health and illness are related to the basic, culture-bound values by which we define a given experience and perception.[1]

Fejos describes culture as "the sum total of socially inherited characteristics of a human group that comprises everything which one generation can tell, convey, or hand down to the next; in other words, the non-physically inherited traits we possess."[2] Another way of understanding the concept of culture is to picture it as the "luggage" that each of us carries around for our lifetime. It is the sum of beliefs, practices, habits, likes, dislikes, norms, customs, rituals, and so forth that we have learned from our families during the years of socialization. In turn, we transmit cultural "luggage" to our own children. The society is which we live—and other forces such as political, economic, and social— tend to alter the way in which some aspects of a particular culture are transmitted and maintained. However, many of the essential components of a given culture do pass from one generation to the next unaltered. Consequently, much of what we believe, think, and do, both consciously and unconsciously, is determined by our cultural background. In this way, culture and ethnicity are handed down from one generation to another.

CULTURE AND ETHNICITY

Cultural background is a fundamental component of one's ethnic background. At this point, a definition of operational terms is called for so that we can proceed from the same point of reference:[3]

> Ethnic: adj. 1. of or pertaining to a social group within a cultural and social system that claims or is accorded special status on the basis of complex, often variable traits including religious, linguistic, ancestral, or physical characteristics. 2. Broadly, characteristic of a religious, racial, national, or cultural group. 3. Pertaining to a people not Christian or Jewish; heathen; pagan: "These Are Ancient Ethnic Revels of a Faith Long Since Forsaken." (Longfellow)

The term *ethnic* has for some time aroused strongly negative feelings and is often rejected by the general population. One can speculate that reasons for the upsurge in the use of the term are the recent interest of people in discovering their personal backgrounds, as well as appeals that politicians have made when they overtly court "the ethnics." Paradoxically, in a nation as large and comprised of as many different peoples as is the United States—with the American Indians being the only true native population—we find ourselves still reluctant to speak of ethnicity and ethnic differences. This stance stems from the fact that most foreign groups that came to this land have more often shed the ways of the "old country" and quickly attempted to assimilate themselves into the mainstream, or the so-called melting pot.[4]

Therefore we need to clarify other operational terms that will occur in this discussion: [5,6]

> **Ethnicity:** n. 1. The condition of belonging to a particular ethnic group. 2. Ethnic pride.
>
> **Ethnocentrism:** n. 1. Belief in the superiority of one's own ethnic group. 2. Overriding concern with race.
>
> **Xenophobe:** n. A person unduly fearful or contemptuous of strangers or foreigners, especially as reflected in his political or cultural views.
>
> **Xenophobia:** A morbid fear of strangers.

The behavorial manifestations of these phenomena occur in response to people's needs, especially when they are foreign born and must find a way to function (1) before they are assimilated into the mainstream and (2) in order to accept themselves. These people cluster together against the majority, who in turn may be discriminating against them.

The United States was once considered a "melting pot" of diverse ethnic and cultural groups. One aspect of the American dream was that all of these diverse groups would blend and assimilate into one common whole. This did not really occur, and today there are many groups that cling to and identify with their ethnic heritage. In fact, among the third-, fourth-, or in some cases subsequent-generation Americans, there are those who desire to know where they come from (who they are). The phenomenon of seeking one's heritage is widespread in today's society:[7] a fine example of this is Alex Haley's book and movie, which documents his search for his family's *Roots*.

Because the "melting pot"—which carried with it the dream of assimilation into a common culture—has proved to be a myth and faded, it is now time to identify and both accept and appreciate the differences among people. It is suggested that this be done not to change people so that they are all alike, but to better understand both one's own ethnic culture and the ethnic culture of other people living in this society. Within the health professions, this is mandatory: because health-care providers learn from their culture the why and the how of being healthy or ill, it behooves them to treat each client with deference to his own cultural background.

In a population that is socialized into a given culture and sub-sequently resocialized into what I define as the *provider culture,* one deals in intimate contact with people who may choose to maintain their traditional perceptions and beliefs regarding health and illness. Here lies the paradox: one culture may believe, for example, that people should starve a cold and feed a fever; another may believe the opposite. Thus there are "elopements" from clinics, broken appointments, and failures to follow prescribed regimens.

THE PROVIDER CULTURE

The providers of health care—physicians, nurses, social workers, dietitians, laboratory and departmental professionals, and so forth—are socialized into the "culture" of their profession. Pro-fessional socialization teaches the student a set of beliefs, prac-tices, habits, likes, dislikes, norms, and rituals (components already described as factors that comprise a given culture). This newly learned information regarding health and illness differs to varying degrees from that of the individual's initial background. As students become more and more knowledgeable, they usually move farther and farther from their past belief systems and, in-deed, farther from the population at large in terms of its under-standing and beliefs regarding health and illness. How often people have stated: "I have no idea what the nurses and doctor are saying!" "They speak a foreign language!" "What they are doing is so strange to me."

In light of the ideas just advanced, health-care providers can be viewed as comprising a foreign culture or ethnic group. They have a social and cultural system; they experience "ethnicity" in the way that they perceive themselves in relation to the health-care consumer. Even if they deny the reality of the situation, health-care providers must understand that they are ethnocentric. Not only are they ethnocentric, but many of them are also xenophobic. In order to appreciate this critical issue, one must consider the following. A principal reason that there is often such difficulty experienced between the health-care provider and the consumer is that health-care providers, with few exceptions, adhere rigidly to the Western system of health-care delivery. With few exceptions they do not publicly sanction any methods of prevention or healing other than "scientifically proved" ones. They ordinarily fail to recognize or use any sources of medication other than those that have been "proved" to be effective by scientific means. The only types of healers that are sanctioned are those that have been educated and certified according to the requirements of this culture.

What happens, then, when people of one belief system encounter people who have other beliefs regarding health and illness (either in prevention or in treatment)? Is the provider able to meet the needs as perceived and defined by the patient? More often than not, there is a wall of misunderstanding between the two. At this point, there occurs what is commonly referred to as a "breakdown in communications"—and we know who ends up on the short end of the situation: the *consumer*.

Providers think that they comprehend all facets of health and illness. Granting that, by training and education, they are at a significant distance from the consumer-patient, I nevertheless suggest and *insist* that it is entirely appropriate for them to explore alternative ideas regarding health and illness and to adjust their approach to coincide with the needs of the specific client. In the past, health-care providers have tried to force Western medicine on one and all, come what may. It is time that health care coincided with the needs of the client instead of inducing additional conflict.

The following list documents the more obvious aspects of the health-care provider's culture. In connection with later chapters, it can be referred to as a framework of comparison with various other ethnic and cultural beliefs and practices.

The Health-Care Provider's Culture

1. Beliefs
   a. Standardized definitions of health and illness.
   b. The omnipotence of technology.
2. Practices
   a. The maintenance of health and the prevention of disease via such mechanisms as the avoidance of stress and the use of immunizations.

      b. Annual physical examinations and diagnostic procedures such as Pap smears.

3. Habits
      a. Charting.
      b. The constant use of jargon.
      c. Use of a systematic approach and problem-solving methodology.

4. Likes
      a. Promptness.
      b. Neatness and organization.
      c. Compliance.

5. Dislikes
      a. Tardiness.
      b. Disorderliness and disorganization.

6. Customs
      a. Professional deference and adherence to the "pecking order" found in autocratic and bureaucratic systems.
      b. "Hand-washing."
      c. Employment of certain procedures attending birth and death.

7. Rituals
      a. The physical examination.
      b. The surgical procedure.
      c. Limiting visitors and visiting hours.

Epidemiology

Another area in which culture plays a broad role is in the interpretation of the causation of illness, or *epidemiology*. The science is inherent in the health-care educational process. In the study of epidemiology, the relationships among the host, agent, and environment are explored. The modern approach attributes the cause of disease (the agent) to bacteria, viruses, chemical carcinogens, pollutants, and so forth. The disorders have names such as pneumonia, meningitis, influenza, polycystic kidney disease, and so on. Unless the student delves further into study of the field, he may well never become familiar with more primitive theories of epidemiology. For example, the concepts of "soul loss," "spirit possession," and "spells" are rarely, if ever, described and discussed during the educational process of health-care providers.[8] Yet these phenomena, too, contribute to people's perceptions of the cause of a given disease.

I have found many students who were familiar with concepts such as "evil eye," and in some instances they took precautions to protect themselves. As discussed in an earlier chapter, they often were forced to take these precautions because of the beliefs of their mothers or grandmothers. After much thought, the acquisition of new facts, and further learning experiences, many of the students chose to shed such beliefs and not *consciously* practice what they had been taught by their families. However, others admitted to still holding such beliefs—but constantly experiencing conflict. This group of students can be viewed as a microcosm of the larger society. It is known that there are many people who cling to familiar belief systems, a fact that lends comfort to them. (In what other way can some of the hardships of life be explained in a more satisfactory or acceptable manner?)

Another facet of epidemiology that one does not ordinarily encounter in academia is that of the causative agent's being another person and not a microbe. The idea of another person's making someone ill by the use of witchcraft or voodoo (or some other form of magic) is unusual content matter within the constraints of a traditional curriculum. However, if the student is to study the cultural perceptions of health and illness, some knowledge of a belief in magic is important. The environment that fosters the use of these agents is one in which hate, envy, and/or jealousy may exist. The way of preventing illness thus caused involves not provoking the wrath of one's friends, neighbors, and enemies. A victim of disease may believe that his success provoked the envy of his friends, that it called the attention of a "witch" to him, or that someone was jealous of a new possession and put a "hex" on him. In the minds of people who still believe and practice so-called primitive health beliefs, these contributing factors are as real as the bacteria and viruses of modern epidemiology are to health-care providers. Regardless of his own belief system, the provider needs to keep an open mind if he is to provide *useful* care to consumers who retain primitive beliefs.

ETHNIC VARIATIONS IN RESPONSE TO PAIN

"Mr. Smith in room 222 is the ideal patient. He never has a single complaint of pain."

"Mrs. Cohen in room 223 is a real complainer. She is constantly asking for pain medication and putting on her light."

"Mrs. O'Mally in room 224 is an ideal patient. She never complains about pain. For that matter, she never complains."

"Mr. Chen in room 225 says nothing. I often wonder what he is feeling."

"Mrs. Petrini in room 226 dramatically cries every time I look at her and complains of pain at every opportunity."

The above statements (however stereotypic) are descriptions of behaviors observed concerning patients' responses to the subjective feeling of pain. Social scientists, health-care researchers, and other professionals maintain that the phenomenon is culture bound: how pain and discomfort—or, for that matter, most emotions—are presented varies among cultures. A person raised in one cultural background may be allowed the free and open expression of his feelings, whereas a person from another culture may have been taught that (for a multitude of reasons) he must never reveal his true feelings.

Let us say that the above statements were all made by the same nurse. Let us go one step further and say that each patient had the same operation on the same day. It would not be, within the limits of general expectations, unusual to see the different patients from differing cultures and ethnic groups exhibit the behaviors described. The fact that culture plans a role in behavior during illness was aptly demonstrated and strongly documented by Mark Zborowski in his study on pain. Briefly, his findings were that Jewish and Italian patients generally responded to pain in an emotional fashion, and they tended to exaggerate the response; "old American Yankees" tended to be more stoic; and the Irish tended to ignore pain.[9,10] Presentation of this type of data can often lead to a major problem: *stereotyping*. Thus I want strongly to emphasize that such descriptions are *general*; the results of one study do not indicate a universal truth. However, even within my own clinical experiences, I have observed events such as those described by the quotations. It is preferable to include and discuss such material rather than to ignore it—particularly inasmuch as there are numerous studies in anthropology, sociology, psychology, and social psychology to support these data, such as findings reported by David Mechanic[11] in 1963 and by Edward Suchman[12,13] in 1964 and 1965.

An abridged article by Irving Zola, which follows the References section, is included in this chapter because it aptly demonstrates many of the points alluded to. Furthermore, it suggests the type of research and analysis that is going on in the field of medical sociology and hence is relevant to any discussion of ethnicity and culture.

REFERENCES

1. Jules Henry, *Culture against Man* (New York: Random House, 1963), p. 323; Eric Bermann, *Scapegoat—The Impact of Death-fear on an American Family* (Ann Arbor: The University of Michigan Press, 1973), pp. 2-4.
2. Paul Fejos, "Man, Magic, and Medicine," in *Medicine and Anthropology*, Iago Goldston, ed. (New York: International University Press, 1959), p. 43.
3. *American Heritage Dictionary of the English Language:* s.v. "ethnic."
4. Michael Novak, "How American Are You If Your Grandparents Came from Serbia in 1888?", in *The Rediscovery of Ethnicity: Its Implications for Culture and Politics in America,* Sallie Te Selle, (ed. New York: Harper and Row, 1973).
5. *American Heritage Dictionary*: s.v. "ethnicity," "ethnocentrism," "xenophobe."
6. Clarince Senior, *The Puerto Ricans: Strangers Then Neighbors.* (Chicago: Quandrangle Books, 1965), p. 21.
7. Sallie Te Selle, ed. *Rediscovery of Ethnicity: Its Implications for Culture and Politics in America.* (New York: Harper and Row, 1973).
8. Irving Kenneth Zola, "The Concept of Trouble and Sources of Medical Assistance: To Whom One Can Turn, with What and Why," *Social Science and Medicine* 6 (1972): 673-679.
9. Mark Zborowski, "Cultural Components in Responses to Pain," *Journal of Social Issues* 8 (1952): 16-30.
10. Mark Zborowski, *People in Pain* (San Francisco: Jossey-Bass, 1969).
11. David Mechanic, "Religion, Religiosity, and Illness Behavior: The Special Case of the Jews," *Human Organization* 22 (1963): 202-208.
12. Edward A. Suchman, "Sociomedical Variations Among Ethnic Groups," *American Journal of Sociology* 70 (1964): 319-331.
13. Edward A. Suchman, "Social Patterns of Illness and Medical Care," *Journal of Health and Human Behavior* 6 (1965): 2-16.

Culture and Symptoms— An Analysis of Patients Presenting Complaints

Irving Kenneth Zola

In most epidemiologic studies, the definition of disease is taken for granted. Yet today's chronic disorders do not lend themselves to such easy conceptualization and measurement as did the contagious disorders of yesteryear. We have long assumed that what constitutes disease is a settled matter, an assumption arising from the tremendous medical and surgical advances of the past half-century. After the current battles against cancer, heart disease, cystic fibrosis, and the like have been won, utopia—a world without disease—will seem right around the corner. Yet after each battle a new enemy seems to emerge. So often has this been the pattern that some have wondered whether life without disease is attainable.

Usually the issue of life without disease has been dismissed as a philosophical problem, a dismissal made considerably easier by our general ideas about the statistical distribution of disorder. For although there is a grudging recognition that each of us must die sometime, illness is generally assumed to be a relatively infrequent, unusual, or abnormal phenomenon. Moreover, the general kinds of

This subchapter is largely based upon an original article that appeared in *American Sociological Review* 31 (October 1966): 615-630.

statistics used to describe illness support such a supposition. Specifically diagnosed conditions, days out of work, and physician visits do occur relatively infrequently for most of us. Although such statistics represent only treated illness, we rarely question whether such data give a true picture. Implicit is the further notion that people who no not consult physicians and other medical agencies (and thus do not appear in the "illness" statistics) may be regarded as healthy.

Yet studies have increasingly appeared which note the large number of disorders that escape detection. Whether based on physicians' estimates[1] or on the recall of lay populations,[2] the proportion of untreated disorders amounts to two-thirds or three-fourths of all existing conditions. The most reliable data, however, come from periodic health examinations and community "health" surveys.[3] At least two such studies noted that as many as 90 percent of the apparently healthy people in their sample had some physical aberration or clinical disorder.[4] Moreover, neither the type of disorder nor the seriousness by objective medical standards differentiated those who felt sick from those who did not. In one of the studies, only 40 percent of those who felt sick were under medical care.[5] It seems that the more intensive the investigation, the higher the prevalence of clinically serious but previously undiagnosed and untreated disorders.

Such data as these give an unexpected statistical picture of illness.* Instead of sickness being a relatively infrequent or abnormal phenomenon, empirical reality suggests that illness—defined as the presence of clinically serious symptoms—is the statistical *norm*.[6] What is particularly striking about this line of reasoning is that the statistical notions underlying many "social" pathologies are similarly being questioned. A number of social scientists have noted that certain deviations—such as lawbreaking, addictive behaviors, sexual "perversions," or mental illness—

---

*Consider the following computation of Hinkle *et al.*[6] They noted that the average lower-middle-class male between the ages of 20 and 45 experiences over a 20-year period approximately 1 life-endangering illness, 20 disabling illnesses, 200 nondisabling illnesses, and 1000 symptomatic episodes. These figures total 1221 sicknesses over 7305 days, or 1 new episode every 6 days. And this takes no account of the duration of a particular condition, nor does it consider any disorder of which the respondent may be unaware. In short, even among a supposedly "healthy" population, scarcely a day goes by wherein people would not be able to report a symptomatic experience.

occur so frequently in the population that if one were to tabulate all the deviations that people possess or engage in, virtually no one could escape the label of "deviant."

Why are so relatively few potential "deviants" labeled such or, more accurately, why do so few come to the attention of official agencies? Perhaps the focus on how or why a particular deviation arose in the first place might be misplaced; an equally important issue for research might be the individual and societal reaction to the deviation once it occurs. Might it then be the differential response to deviation rather than the prevalence of the deviation that accounts for many reported group and subgroup differences?

A similar set of questions can be asked with regard to physical illness. Given that the prevalence of clinical abnormalities is so high and the rate of acknowledgement so low, how representative are the "treated" of all those with a particular condition? Given further that what *is* treated seems unrelated to what would usually be thought to be the objective situation—i.e., seriousness, degree of disability, and subjective discomfort—is it possible that some selective process is operating in what gets counted or tabulated as illness?

THE INTERPLAY OF CULTURE AND "SYMPTOMS"

Holding in abeyance the idea that many epidemiologic differences may in fact be due to as yet undiscovered etiologic forces, we may speculate on how such differences come to exist or on how a selective process of attention may operate. Upon surveying many cross-cultural comparisons of morbidity, we concluded that there are at least two ways in which signs ordinarily defined as indicating problems in one population may be ignored in others. The first is related to the actual prevalence of the sign, and the second to its congruence with dominant or major value orientations.

In the first instance, when the aberration is fairly widespread, this in itself might constitute a reason for its not being considered "symptomatic" or unusual. Among many Mexican-Americans in the southwestern United States, diarrhea, sweating, and coughing are everyday experiences;[7] among certain groups of Greeks, trachoma is almost universal.[8] Even within our own society,

Koos has noted that, although low-back pain is quite a common condition among lower-class women, it is not considered symptomatic of any disease or disorder but part of their expected everyday existence.[9] For the population in which the particular condition is ubiquitous, the condition is perceived as the normal state.[10] This does not mean that it is considered "good" (although instances have been noted in which not having the endemic condition was considered abnormal*), but rather that it is natural and inevitable and thus to be ignored as being of no consequence. Because the "symptoms" or conditions are omnipresent (they always were and always will be), there exists for such populations or cultures simply no frame of reference by which these symptoms could be considered a deviation.

In the second process, it is the "fit" of certain signs with a society's major values that accounts for the degree of attention they receive. For example, in some nonliterate societies there is anxiety-free acceptance of and willingness to describe hallucinatory experiences. Wallace noted that in such societies the fact of hallucination *per se* is seldom disturbing; its content is the focus of interest. In Western society, however, with its emphasis on rationality and control, the very admission of hallucinations is commonly taken to be a grave sign and, in some literature, regarded as the essential feature of psychosis.[11] In such instances, it is not the sign itself or its frequency that is significant but the social context within which it occurs and within which it is perceived and understood. Even more explicit workings of this process can be seen in the interplay of "symptoms" and social roles. Tiredness, for example, is a physical sign that is not only ubiquitous but a correlate of a vast number of disorders. Yet among a group of my students who kept a diary in which they noted all bodily states and conditions, tiredness, although often recorded, was rarely cited as a cause for concern. Attending school and being among peers who stressed the importance of hard work and achievement, almost as an end in itself, the students regarded tiredness not as an indication of something wrong but as positive proof that they were doing right. If they were tired, it must be because they had

*For example, Ackerknecht[10] noted that pinto (dichromic spirochetosis), a skin disease, was so common among some South American tribes that the few single men who were not suffering from it were regarded as pathologic to the degree of being excluded from marriage.

been working hard. In such a setting, tiredness would rarely in itself be either a cause for concern and regarded as a symptom or reason for action or seeking medical aid.[12]

Also illustrative of this process are the divergent perceptions of those bodily complaints often referred to as "female troubles."[13] Nausea is a common and treatable concomitant of pregnancy, yet Margaret Mead records no morning sickness among the Arapesh. Her data suggest that this may be related to the almost complete denial that a child exists, until shortly before birth.[14] In a Christian setting, in which the existence of life is dated from conception, nausea becomes the external sign, hope, and proof that one is pregnant. Thus, in the United States, this symptom not only is quite widespread but is also an expected and almost welcome part of pregnancy. A quite similar phenomenon is the recognition of dysmenorrhea. While Arapesh women reported no pain during menstruation,* quite the contrary is reported in the United States.[15] Interestingly enough, the only consistent factor related to dysmenorrhea's occurence among American women was a learning one—those who experienced it reported having observed its manifestations in other women during their childhood.†[16-18]

From examples such as these, it seems likely that the degree of recognition and treatment of certain gynecologic problems may be traced to the prevailing definition of what constitutes a necessary part of the business of being a women. That such divergent definitions are still operative is shown by two recent

---

*Mead does note that this lack of perception, as far as the Arapesh are concerned, may be related to the considerable self-induced discomfort prescribed for women during menstruation.

†The fact that one has to learn that something is painful or unpleasant has been noted elsewhere. Mead reports that in causalgia a given individual suffers and reports pain because she is *aware* of uterine contractions and not because of the occurrence of these contractions. Others studying addictive behaviors (e.g., Becker[17]) have noted not only that an individual has to learn that the experience is pleasurable but also that a key factor in becoming addicted is the recognition of the association of withdrawal symptoms with the lack of drugs. Medical patients who had been heavily dosed and then withdrawn, even though they experience symptoms as a result of withdrawal, may attribute them to their general convalescent aches and pains. Schacter and Singer[18] reported a series of experiments in which epinephrine-injected subjects defined their mood as euphoria or anger depending on whether they spent time with a euphoric or angry stooge. Subjects without injections reported no such change in mood responding to these same social situations. This led Schacter and Singer to the contention that the diversity of human emotional experiences stems from differential labeling of similar physical sensations.

studies. In the first, 78 mothers of lower socioeconomic status were required to keep health calendars over a four-week period. Despite the instruction to report *all* bodily states and dysfunctions, only 14 even *noted* the occurrence of menses or its accompaniment.[19] A second study, done on a higher socioeconomic group, yielded a different expression of the same phenomenon. Over a period of several years, the author collected four-week health calendars from students. The women in the sample had at least a college education and virtually all were committed to careers in the behavioral sciences. Within this group there was little failure to report menses; very often medication was taken for the discomforts of dysmenorrhea. Moreover, this group was so psychologically sophisticated or self-conscious that they interpreted or questioned most physical signs or symptoms as attributable to some psychosocial stress. There was only one exception: dysmenorrhea. Thus, even in this "culturally advantaged" group, the disorder was interpreted as a sign of a *bodily* condition and not subjected to psychologic analysis.

In the opening section of this paper, we presented evidence that a selective process might well be operating in what symptoms are brought to the attention of a physician. We also noted that it might be this selective process and not an etiologic one that accounts for the many unexplained or overexplained epidemiologic differences observed among and within societies. (There may even be no "real" differences in the prevalence rates of many deviations.* Such selective processes are probably present at all the stages through which an individual and his condition must pass before he ultimately gets counted as "ill." In this section we have focused on one of these stages, the perception of a particular bodily state as a symptom, and have delineated two possible ways in which the culture or social setting might influence the awareness of something as abnormal and thus its eventual tabulation in medical statistics.

---

*For example, a study of peptic-ulcer incidence in African tribal groups[20] first confirmed the stereotype that it was relatively infrequent among such groups and therefore that it was associated (as many had claimed) with the stresses and strains of modern living. Yet when he relied not on reported diagnosis but on autopsy data, he found that the scars of peptic ulcer were no less common than in Britain. He concluded, "There is no need to assume that in backward communities peptic ulcer does not develop; it is only more likely to go undetected because the conditions that might bring it to notice do not exist."

SAMPLE SELECTION AND METHODOLOGY

In previous research the specific method of measuring and studying symptoms has varied among case-record analysis, symptom
checklists, and interviews. The data have been either retrospective
or projective, that is, requesting the subject either to recall symptoms experienced during a specific time period or to choose symptoms that would bother him sufficiently to seek medical aid.
Such procedures do not provide data on the complaints that
people actually bring to a physician, a fact of particular importance
in light of the many investigations that point to the lack of, and
distortions in, recall of sickness episodes. An equally serious
problem is the effect of what the physician, medicine man, or
health expert may tell the patient about the latter's subsequent
perceptions of and recall of his ailment. We resolved these problems
by restricting the sample to new patients on their first medical
visit to the clinics and by interviewing them during the waiting
period *before* they were seen by a physician.

The primary method of data collection was a focused, open-
ended interview dealing with the patient's own or family's
responses to his presenting complaints. Interspersed throughout
the interview were a number of more objective measures of
the patient's responses—checklists, forced-choice comparisons,
attitudinal items, and scales. Other information included a
demographic background questionnaire, a review of the medical
record, and a series of ratings by each patient's examining physician as to the primary diagnosis, the secondary diagnosis, the
potential seriousness, and the degree of clinical urgency (i.e., the
necessity that the patient be seen immediately) of the patient's
presenting complaint.

THE PATIENT AND HIS ILLNESS

The data are based on a comparison between 63 Italians (34
female, 29 male) and 81 Irish (42 female, 39 male) who were new
admissions to the EENT and medical clinics of the Massachusetts
General Hospital and the Massachusetts Eye and Ear Infirmary
and who were seen between July 1960 and February 1961. The
mean age of each ethnic group (male and female computed sep-

arately) was approximately 33. Although most patients were married, there was, in the sample, a higher proportion of single Irish men—a finding of other studies involving the Irish[21] and not unexpected from our knowledge of Irish family structure.[22] Most respondents had between 10 and 12 years of schooling, but only about 30 percent of the males claimed to have graduated from high school as compared with nearly 60 percent of the females. There were no significant differences on standard measures of social class, although in education, social class, occupation of the breadwinner in the patient's family, and occupation of the patient's father, the Irish ranked slightly higher. The Italians were over-whelmingly American-born children of foreign parents; about 80 percent were second generation, and 20 percent were third. Among the Irish about 40 percent were second generation, 30 percent third, and 30 percent fourth.

With regard to general medical coverage, there were no clear differences between the ethnic groups. Approximately 62 percent of the sample had health insurance, a figure similar to the comparable economic group in the Rosenfeld survey of Metropolitan Boston.[23] In our sample, 60 percent had physicians whom they would call family physicians. The Irish tended more than the Italians to perceive themselves as having poor health, claiming more often that they had been seriously ill in the past. This was consistent with their reporting of the most recent visit to a physician: nine of the Irish but none of the Italians claimed to have had a recent major operation (e.g., appendectomy) or illness (e.g., pneumonia). Although there were no differences in the actual seriousness of their present disorders (according to the physician's ratings), there was a tendency for the examining physician to consider the Irish as being in more urgent need of treatment. It was evident that the patients were not in the throes of an acute illness, although they may have been experiencing an acute episode. There was a light tendency for the Irish, as a group, to have had their complaints longer. More significantly, the women of both groups claimed to have borne their symptoms for a longer time than the men.

In confining the study to three clinics, we were trying not only to economize but also to limit the range of illnesses. The latter was necessary for investigating differential responses to essentially similar conditions. Yet, at best, this is only an approximate control. To resolve this difficulty, after all initial comparisons were made between the ethnic groups as a whole, the data were examined for a selected subsample with a specific control for diagnosis. This subsample consisted of matched pairs of one Irish and one Italian of the same sex, who had the same primary diagnosis and whose disorder was of approximately the same duration and rated (by the examining physician) as similar in degree of "seriousness." Wherever numbers made it feasible, there was a further matching on age, marital status, and education. In all, 37 diagnostically matched pairs (18 females and 19 males) were created; these constituted the final test of any findings of the differential response to illness.*

LOCATION AND QUALITY OF PRESENTING COMPLAINTS

In the folklore of medical practice, the supposed opening question is: "Where does it hurt?" This query provides the starting point of our analysis—the perceived location of the patient's troubles. Our first finding (Table R.1) is that more Irish than Italians tended to locate their chief problem in either the eye, the ear, the nose, or the throat (and more so for females than for males). The same tendency was evident when all patients were asked what they considered to be the most important part of their body and the one with which they would be most concerned if something went wrong (Table R.2). Here, too, significantly more Irish emphasized difficulties of the eye, the ear, the nose, or the throat. We doubt that this reflected merely a difference in the conditions for which they were seeking aid because the two other parts of the body most frequently referred to were heart and "mind" locations, and these represent only 3 percent of the primary diagnoses of the entire sample. In the retesting of these findings on diagnostically matched pairs, although there were a great many ties, the general directions were still consistent. Thus, even when Italians had a diagnosed eye or ear disorder, they did

*These pairs included some 18 distinct diagnoses: conjunctivitis, eyelid disease (e.g., blepharitis), myopia, hyperopia, vitreous opacities, impacted cerumen, external otitis, otitis media, otosclerosis, deviated septum, sinusitis, nasopharyngitis, allergy, thyroid conditions, obesity, functional complaints, no pathology, psychological problems.

Table R.1. Distribution of Irish and Italian Clinic Admission by Location of Chief Complaint

Location of Complaint	Italian	Irish*
Eye, ear, nose, or throat	34	61
Other parts of the body	29	17
Total	63	78

*Since three Irish patients (two women, one man) claimed to be asymptomatic, no location could be determined from their viewpoint.

Note: $\chi^2 = 9.31$; $p < 0.01$.

not locate their chief complaints there, nor did they focus their future concern on these locations.

Pain, the most common accompaniment of illness, was the dimension of patients' symptoms to which we next turned. Pain is an especially interesting phenomenon as there is considerable evidence that its tolerance and perception are not purely physiologic responses and do not necessarily reflect the degree of objective discomfort induced by a particular disorder or experimental procedure. In our study not only did the Irish more often than the Italians deny that pain was a feature of their illness, but this difference held even for those patients with the same disorder (Table R.3). When the Irish were asked directly about the

Table R.2. Distribution of Irish and Italian Clinic Admission by Part of the Body Considered Most Important

Most Important Part of the Body	Italian	Irish
Eye, ear, nose, or throat	6	26
Other parts of the body	57	55
Total	63	81

Note: $\chi^2 = 10.50$; $p < 0.01$.

Table R.3. Distribution of Irish and Italian Clinic Admission by Presence of Pain in Their Current Illness

Presence of Pain	Italian	Irish
No	27	54
Yes	36	27
Total	63	81

Note: χ^2 = 10.26; $p < 0.01$.

presence of pain, some hedged their replies with qualifications: "It was more a throbbing than a pain . . . not really pain, it feels more like sand in my eye." Such comments indicated that the patients were reflecting something more than an objective reaction to their physical conditions.

Although there were no marked differences in the length, frequency, or outward manifestation of their symptoms, a difference did emerge in the ways in which these subjects described the quality of the physical difficulty embodied in their chief complaint (Table R.4). Two types of difficulty were distinguished: one was of a more limited nature and emphasized a circumscribed and specific dysfunctioning; the second emphasized a difficulty of a grosser and more diffuse quality.* When the patients' complaints were analyzed according to these two types, proportionately more Irish described their chief problem in terms of specific dysfunction, whereas proportionately more Italians spoke of a diffuse difficulty. Once again, the findings for diagnostically matched pairs were in the predicted direction.

This difference was further demonstrated in two independent ways—the total number of parts and functions that the patient claimed were affected and the degree to which the patient felt his/her illness disrupted his/her social relationships. Thus, compared with the Irish, the Italians presented significantly more

*Complaints of the first type emphasized a somewhat limited difficulty and dysfunction best exemplified by something specific, e.g., an organ's having gone wrong in a particular way. The second type seemed to involve a more attenuated kind of problem the location and scope of which were less determinate and the description of which was finally more qualitative and less measurable.

Table R.4. Distribution of Irish and Italian Clinic Admissions by Quality of Physical Difficulty Embodied in Chief Complaints

Quality of Physical Difficulty	Italian	Irish*
Problems of a diffuse nature	43	33
Problems of a specific nature	20	45
Total	63	78

*Since three Irish patients (two women, one man) claimed to be asymptomatic, no rating of the quality of physical difficulty could be determined from their viewpoint.

Note: $\chi^2 = 9.44$; $p < 0.01$.

symptoms, had symptoms in more bodily locations, and noted more types of bodily dysfunctions. Similarly, the Italians complained of being irritable and feeling that their symptoms affected their daily lives, whereas the Irish consistently denied any such effect.

Table R.5 offers a final illustration of how differently these patients reacted to and perceived their illnesses. Each set of responses was given by an Italian and an Irish patient of similar age and sex with a disorder of approximately the same duration and with the same primary and secondary diagnosis (if there was one). In the first two cases, the Irish patient focused on a specific malfunctioning as the main concern, whereas the Italian did not even mention this aspect of the problem but went on to describe more diffuse qualities of his condition. The last four responses contrast the Italian and Irish answers to questions about pain and interpersonal relations.

SOCIOCULTURAL COMMUNICATION

In theorizing about the interplay of culture and symptoms, we gave particular emphasis to the "fit" of certain bodily states with dominant value orientations. The empirical examples for the latter were drawn primarily from data on social roles. Of course,

Table R.5. Differences between Italians and Irish in Their Responses to and Perceptions of Their Illnesses

Diagnosis	Question of Interviewer	Irish Patient	Italian Patient
1. Presbyopia and hyperopia	What seems to be the trouble?	I can't seem to thread a needle or read a paper.	I have a constant headache, and my eyes seem to get all red and burny.
	Anything else?	No, I can't recall any.	No, just that it lasts all day long and I even wake up with it sometimes.
2. Myopia	What seems to be the trouble?	I can't see across the street.	My eyes seem very burny, especially the right eye. Two or three months ago I woke up with my eyes swollen. I bathed it and it did go away, but there was still the burny sensation.
	Anything else?	I had been experiencing headaches, but it may be that I'm in early menopause.	Yes, there always seems to be a red spot beneath this eye . . . .
	Anything else?	No.	Well, my eyes feel very heavy. . . . at night they bother me most.

3. Otitis externa A.D.	Is there any pain?	There's a congestion . . . but it's a pressure, not really a pain.	Yes . . . if I rub it, it disappears . . . I had a pain from my shoulder up to my neck and thought it might be a cold.
4. Pharyngitis	Is there any pain?	No, maybe a slight headache but nothing that lasts.	Yes, I have had a headache a few days. Oh, yes, every time I swallow it's annoying.
5. Presbyopia and hyperopia	Do you think the symptoms affected how you got along with your family? your friends?	No, I have had loads of trouble. I can't imagine this bothering me.	Yes, when I have a headache, I'm very irritable, very tense, very short-tempered.
6. Deafness, hearing loss	Did you become irritable?	No, not me . . . maybe everybody else, but not me.	Oh, yes . . . the least little thing aggravates me . . . and I take it out on the children.

values are evident on even more general levels—such as formal and informal societal sanctions and the culture's orientation to life's basic problems. With an orientation to problems usually goes a preferred solution or way of handling them. Thus a society's values may also be reflected in such preferred solutions. One behavioral manifestation of this is in the defense mechanism: a part of the everyday way individuals have of dealing with their everyday stresses and strains. We contend that illness and its treatment (from taking medicine to seeing a physician) are one of these everyday stresses and strains: an anxiety-laden situation[24] that calls forth coping or defense mechanisms. From this general reasoning, we would thus speculate that Italian and Irish ways of communicating illness may reflect major values and preferred ways of handling problems within the culture itself.

For the Italians, the large number of symptoms and the spread of the complaints—not only throughout the body but with respect to other aspects of life—may be understood in terms of their expressiveness and expansiveness, qualities described so often in sociologic, historical, and fictional writing. And yet their illness behavior seems to reflect something more than lack of inhibition and valuation of spontaneity. There is something larger than life in their behavior: a well-seasoned, dramatic emphasis. In fact, clinicians have noted that this openness is deceptive; it goes only so far. Thus the Italian overstatement of "symptoms" is not merely an expressive quality but perhaps a more general mechanism, a special way of handling problems—a defense mechanism we call dramatization. Dynamically, dramatization seems to allow one to cope with anxiety by repeating it. Anne Parsons[25] delineates this process in a case study of a schizophrenic woman. Through repetition and exaggeration the patient was able to isolate and defend herself from the destructive consequences of her own psychotic breakdown. Parsons concludes:

> . . . rather than appearing as evidence for the greater acceptance of id impulses the greater dramatic expression of Southern Italian culture might be given a particular place among the ego mechanisms, different from but in this respect fulfilling the same function as the emphasis on rational mastery of the objective or subjective world which characterizes our own culture [U.S.A.].[25]

Although other social historians have noted the Italian flair for show and spectacle, Barzini has most explicitly related this phenomenon to the coverup of omnipresent tragedy and poverty, a way of making daily life bearable, the satisfactory *ersatz* for the many things that are lacking.

> The most easily identifiable reasons why the Italians love their own show: ... First of all they do it to tame and prettify savage nature, to make life bearable, dignified, significant and pleasant for others, and themselves. They do it then for their own private ends; a good show makes a man *simpatico* to powerful people, helps him get on in the world and obtain what he wants, solves many problems, lubricates the wheels of society, protects him from the envy of his enemies and the arrogance of the mighty—they do it to avenge themselves on unjust fate.[26]

If dramatization is a valued and preferred way of handling problems, then the experience of illness provides yet another stage.

But if the Italian view of life is expressed through its fiestas, for the Irish it is expressed through its fasts. Their life has been depicted as one of long periods of plodding routine followed by episodes of wild adventure and of lengthy postponement of the gratifications of sex and marriage, interspersed with brief, immediate satisfactions such as fighting and carousing. Perhaps in recognition of the expected and limited nature of such outbursts, the most common Irish outlet, alcoholism, is often referred to as "a good man's weakness." Life is black and long-suffering; the less said the better.*

It is the last statement that best reflects the Irish handling of illness. Whereas in other contexts the ignoring of bodily complaints is merely descriptive of what is going on, in Irish culture it seems to be the prescribed and supported defense mechanism singularly most appropriate for psychological and physical survival.* When speaking of the discomfort caused by her illness, an Irish woman

---

*The ubiquitous comic spirit, humor, and wit for which the Irish are famous can be regarded in part as a functional equivalent of the dramatization used by Italians. It is a cover, a way of isolating life's hardships, and at the same time a preventive of deeper examination and probing.[27] Also, although their daily life was endowed with great restrictions, their fantasy life was replete with great richness (e.g., tales of "wee folk").

stated, "I ignore it like I do most things." In terms of presenting complaints this understatement and restraint were even more evident. They could be seen in the Irish patients' seeming reluctance to admit they had any symptoms at all, in their limiting their symptoms to the specific location in which they arose, and in their contention that their physical problems affected nothing in their lives but the most minute physical functioning. The consistency of this illness behavior with the Irish people's general view of life is shown in two other contexts. First, it helped perpetuate a self-fulfilling prophecy. Thus their way of communicating complaints—although doing little to make treatment easy—did ensure some degree of continual suffering and thus further proof that life is painful and hard (that is, "full of facts").† Second, their illness behavior can be linked to the sin and guilt ideology that seems to pervade so much of Irish society. In a culture where restraint is the *modus operandi*, temptation is ever-present and must be guarded against. As the flesh is weak, there is a concomitant expectation that sin is likely. Thus, when unexpected or unpleasant events take place, the Irish search for what they did or must have done wrong. Perhaps their three most favored locations of symptoms (the eyes, ears, and throat) might be understood as symbolic reflections of the more immediate source of their sin and guilt: what they should not have seen; what they should not have heard; what they should not have said.

In these few paragraphs, we have tried to provide a link between membership in a cultural group and the communication of bodily complaints. The illness behavior of the Irish and the Italians has

*According to Spiegel and Kluckhohn,[28] the Irishman's major avenue of relief from his oppressive sense of guilt lies in his almost unlimited capacity for denial. This capacity they claim is fostered by the perception in the rural Irish of a harmonic blending between man and nature. Such harmonizing of man and nature is further interpreted as blurring the elements of causality, thus allowing for continually shifting the responsibility for events from one person to another, and even from a person to animistically conceived forces. Thus, denial becomes not only a preferred avenue of relief but also one supported and perhaps elicited by their perception of their environment.

†Their "fantasizing" and their "fasting" might be reflected in the serious illness they claim to have had in the past and the dire consequences they forecasted for their future. We do not know for a fact that the Irish had more serious illnesses than the Italians but merely that they claimed to. The Italians might well have had similar conditions but did not necessarily consider them serious.

been explained in terms of two of the more generally prescribed defense mechanisms used in their respective cultures: the Irish handling their troubles by denial and the Italians handling theirs by dramatization.

CONCLUSION

The discerning of reactions to minor problems harks back to a point mentioned in the early pages of this report. Whereas sociologists, anthropologists, and mental-health workers have usually considered sociocultural factors to be etiologic factors in the creation of specific problems, the interpretive emphasis in this study has been on how sociocultural background may lead to different definitions of and responses to essentially the same experience. The strongest evidence in support of this argument is the different ethnic perceptions of what is essentially the same disease. Although it is obvious that not all people react similarly to the same disease process, it is striking that the pattern of response can vary with the ethnic background of the patient. There is little known physiologic difference between ethnic groups that would account for the differing reactions. In fact, the comparison of the matched diagnostic groups led us to believe that, should diagnosis be more precisely controlled, the differences would be even more striking.

The present report has attempted to demonstrate the fruitfulness of an approach that does not take the definition of abnormality for granted. Despite their limitations, our data seem sufficiently striking to provide further reason for reexamining our traditional and often rigid conceptions of health and illness, of normality and abnormality, of conformity and deviance. Symptoms or physical aberrations are so widespread that perhaps relatively few, and a biased selection at best, come to the attention of official treatment agencies such as physicians, hospitals, and public-health agencies. There may even be a sense in which they are part and parcel of the human condition. We have thus tried to present evidence showing that the very labeling and definition of a bodily state as a symptom or as a problem is in itself part of a social process. If there is a selection and definitional process, then focusing solely on the reasons for deviation (i.e., the study of etiology) and ignoring what constitutes a deviation in the eyes of the individual and his society may obscure important aspects of our understanding and eventually our philosophy of treatment and control of illness. Certainly various viewpoints[29] should be considered in our present context.

REFERENCES

1. R.J.F.H. Pinsett, *Morbidity Statistics from General Practice*, Studies of Medical Populations, no. 14 (London: H.M.S.O., 1962); P. Stocks, *Sickness in the Population of England and Wales, 1944-1947*, Studies of Medical Populations, no. 2 (London: H.M.S.O., 1944); John Horder and Elizabeth Horder, "Illness in General Practice," *Practitioner* 173 (August 1954): 177-185.

2. Charles R. Hoffer and Edgar A. Schuler, "Measurement of Health Needs and Health Care," *American Sociological Review* 13 (December 1948): 719-724; Political and Economic Planning, *Family Needs and the Social Services*, (London: Allen and Unwin, 1961); Leonard S. Rosenfeld, Jacob Katz, and Avedis Donabedian, *Medical Care Needs and Services in the Boston Metropolitan Area* (Boston: Medical Care Evaluation Studies, Health, Hospitals, and Medical Care Division, United Community Services of Metropolitan Boston, 1957).

3. Commission on Chronic Illness, *Chronic Illness in a Large City* (Cambridge: Harvard University Press, 1957); J. Wister Meigs, "Occupational Medicine," *New England Journal of Medicine* 264 (April 1961): 861-867; George S. Siegel, *Periodic Health Examinations: Abstracts from the Literature*, Public Health Service Publication 1010 (Washington, D.C.: U.S. Government Printing Office, 1963).

4. Innes H. Pearse and Lucy H. Crocker, *The Peckham Experiment* (London: Allen and Unwin, 1949); *Biologists in Search of Material*, Interim Reports of the Work of the Pioneer Health Center, Peckham (London: Faber and Faber, 1938); Joseph E. Schenthal, "Multiphasic Screening of the Well Patient," *Journal of the American Medical Association* 172 (January 1960): 51-64.

5. Pearse and Crocker, *op cit.*[4]

6. Lawrence E. Hinkle, Jr. et al., "An Examination of the Relation Between Symptoms, Disability, and Serious Illness in Two Homogeneous Groups of Men and Women," *American Journal of Public Health* 50 (September 1960): 1327-1336.

7. Margaret Clark, *Health in the Mexican-American Culture* (Berkeley and Los Angeles: University of California Press, 1958).

8. Richard H. Blum, *The Management of the Doctor-Patient Relationship* (New York: McGraw-Hill, 1960), 11.

9. Earl L. Koos, *The Health of Regionsville* (New York: Columbia University Press, 1954).

10. Erwin W. Ackerknecht, "The Role of Medical History in Medical Education," *Bulletin of History of Medicine* 21 (March-April 1947): 135-145; Allan B. Raper, "The Incidence of Peptic Ulceration in Some African Tribal Groups," *Transactions of the Royal Society of Tropical Medicine and Hygiene:* 152 (November 1958): 535-546.

11. Anthony F.C. Wallace, "Cultural Determinants of Response to Hallucinatory Experience," *Archives of General Psychiatry* 1 (July 1959): 58-69.

12. Barbara L. Carter, "Non-physiological Dimensions of Health and Illness" (unpublished paper, Brandeis University, 1965).

13. Simone de Beauvoir, *The Second Sex* (New York: Knopf, 1957); Helene Deutsch, *The Psychology of Women* (New York: Grune, 1944); Margaret Mead, *Male and Female* (New York: Morrow, 1949).

14. Margaret Mead, *Sex and Temperament in Three Primitive Societies* (New York: Mentor, 1950).

15. Mead, *Male and Female.*[13]

16. Mead, *Male and Female.*[13]

17. Howard S. Becker, *Outsiders* (Glencoe, Ill.: Free Press, 1963).

18. Stanley Schacter and Jerome Singer, "Cognitive, Social, and Physiological Determinants of Emotional State," *Psychological Review* 69 (September 1962): 379-387.

19. John Kosa et al. "Crisis and Family Life: A Re-examination of Concepts," *Wisconsin Sociologist* 4 (Summer 1965): 11-19.

20. Allan B. Raper, *op cit.*[10]

21. Marvin K. Opler and Jerome L. Singer, "Ethnic differences in Behavior and Psychopathology: Italian and Irish,"*International Journal of Social Psychiatry* 2 (Summer 1956): 11-12.

22. Conrad M. Arensberg and Solon T. Kimball, *Family and Community in Ireland* (Cambridge: Harvard University Press, 1948).

23. Rosenfeld, Katz, and Donabedian, *op cit.*[2]

24. Barbara Blackwell, "The Literature of Delay in Seeking Medical Care for Chronic Illnesses," *Health Education Monographs*, no. 16 (1963): 3-32; Bernard Kutner, Henry B. Malcover, and Abraham Oppenheim, "Delay in the Diagnosis and Treatment of Cancer," *Journal of Chronic Diseases* 7 (January 1958): 95-120; Bernard Kutner and Gerald Gordon, "Seeking Aid for Cancer," *Journal of Health and Human Behavior* 2 (Fall 1961): 171-178.

25. Anne Parsons, *Psychiatry*, p. 26.

26. Luigi Barzini, *The Italians* (New York: Bantam Books, 1965), p. 104.

27. Sigmund Freud, *Wit and the Unconscious* (New York: Moffat, Yard, 1916).

28. Spiegel and Kluckhohn, "The Influence of the Family and Cultural Values on the Mental Health and Illness of the Individual." Unpublished progress report of Grant M—971, U.S. Public Health Service.

29. Samuel Butler, *Erewhon* (New York: Signet, 1961); René Dubos, Joseph D. Lohman, and participants, "Juvenile Delinquency: Its Dimensions, Its Conditions, Techniques of Control, Proposals for Action," Subcommittee on Juvenile Delinquency of the Senate Committee on Labor and Public Welfare, 86th Congress, S. 765, S.1090, S. 1314, Spring 1959, p. 268; Talcott Parsons, "Social Change and Medical Organization in the United States: A Sociological Perspective," *Annals of the American Academy of Political and Social Science* 346 (March 1963): 21-34; Edwin M. Schur, *Crimes Without Victims: Deviant Behavior and Public Policy* (Englewood, N.J.: Prentice-Hall, 1965); Thomas Szasz, *The Myth of Mental Illness* (New York: Hoeber-Harper, 1961); Thomas Szasz, *Law, Liberty and Psychiatry* (New York: Macmillan, 1963); Irving Kenneth Zola, "Problems for Research: Some Effects of Assumptions Underlying Socio-Medical Investigations," in *Proceedings, Conference on Medical Sociology and Disease Control,* Gerald Gordon, ed. (National Tuberculosis Association, 1966), pp. 9-17.

BIBLIOGRAPHY: CULTURE, HEALTH, AND ILLNESS

Bermann, Eric. *Scapegoat.* Ann Arbor: University of Michigan Press, 1973.

This book deals not only with the impact of fear of death on an American family, but also with the role of culture in facing this event.

Galdston, Iago, editor. *Medicine and Anthropology.* New York: International Universities Press, 1959.

Excellent background reading, this anthology explores the relation of anthropology to medicine in a number of outstanding articles.

Newman, Katharine D. *Ethnic American Short Stories.* New York: Pocket Books, 1975.

Numerous short stories that depict the literary perceptions and "laws" of various American ethnic groups are presented.

Rude, Donald, editor. *Alienation: Minority Groups.* New York: Wiley, 1972.

> This book explores the values and goals of people who have sought to reshape American society. It examines the paradox in today's society that awards the expression of individuality but casts out those who by race, sex, politics, or mores are "different." It includes essays, poetry, and photography by those who are victims of oppression.

Ryan, William. *Blaming the Victim.* New York: Vintage Books, 1971.

> Ryan demonstrates how the victims of poverty are blamed for their condition rather than the real villain—the inequality of American society.

Te Selle, Sallie, editor. *The Rediscovery of Ethnicity: Its Implications for Culture and Politics in America.* New York: Harper, 1973.

> How "American" are we? This book attempts to answer this question with a number of outstanding contributions by writers such as Michael Novak, Arthur V. Shostack, and Rudolph J. Vecoli.

Zborowski, Mark. *People in Pain.* San Francisco: Jossey-Bass, 1969.

> Zborowski examines feeling of pain as a cultural experience for different peoples with unique histories.

FURTHER SUGGESTED READINGS:

Books

Finney, Joseph C., editor, *Culture Change, Mental Health and Poverty.* New York: Simon and Schuster, 1969.

Landy, David, editor. *Culture, Disease and Healing.* New York: Macmillan, 1977.

Leininger, Madeleine. *Nursing and Anthropology: Two Worlds to Blend.* New York: Wiley, 1970.

Novak, Michael. *The Rise of the Unmeltable Ethnics.* New York: MacMillan, 1971.

Poynter, F. N. L., editor. *Medicine and Culture.* London: Wellcome Institute of the History of Medicine, 1969.

Read, Margaret. *Culture, Health and Disease,* London: Javistock Publications, 1966.

Articles

Blaylock, Jerry. "The Psychological and Cultural Influences on the Reaction to Pain." *Nursing Forum* 7 (1968).

Leininger, Madeleine. "The Cultural Concept and Its Relevance to Nursing."
    Journal of Nursing Education 6 (April 1967): 27.
MacGregor, F. C. "Uncooperative Patients: Some Cultural Interpretations."
    American Journal of Nursing 67 (January 1967): 88-91.
"Symposium on Cultural and Biological Diversity and Health Care." *Nursing
    Clinics of North America* 12 (March 1977): 1.
Zola, Irving Kenneth. "The Concept of Trouble and Sources of Medical
    Assistance: To Whom One Can Turn, With What and Why."
    Social Science and Medicine 6 (1972): 673-679.

CHAPTER 6

Healing

Health-care providers have the opportunity to observe the most incredible phenomenon of life: the recovery from illness. In today's modern society, the healer is the physician, and the other members of the health team all play a significant role in the prevention, detection, and treatment of disease. Yet human beings have existed, some sources suggest, for 2 million years. How, then, did the species *Homo sapiens* survive before the advent of modern technology? It is quite evident that numerous forms of healing existed long before the methodologies that we apply today.

In the natural course of any illness, the stricken individual can expect to experience the following set of events: he becomes ill; the illness may be acute, with concomitant symptoms or signs such as pain, fever, nausea, bleeding, etc. On the other hand, the illness may be insidious, with a gradual progression and worsening of symptoms, which might encompass slow deterioration of movement or an often soul-deadening intensification of pain.

If the illness is mild, the person relies on self-treatment or, as is often the case, does nothing and gradually the symptoms disappear. If the illness is more severe or is of longer duration, the person experiencing the symptoms may consult expert help from a healer of one type or another, usually from a physician.

The person recovers, or expects to recover. As far back as historians and interested social scientists can trace in the history of humankind, this phenomenon of recovery has occurred. In fact, it made very little difference what mode of treatment was used; recovery was usual. It is this occurrence of natural recovery that has given rise to all forms of "healing" that attempt to explain a phenomenon that is natural. That is, one may choose to rationalize the success of a "healing" method by pointing to the patient's recovery. Over the generations, natural healing has been attributed to all sorts of rituals, including trephining, cupping, magic, leeching, and bleeding. From medicine man to sorcerer,[1] the art of healing has passed through succeeding generations. People knew the ailments of their time and devised treatments for them. In spite of ravaging plagues, natural disasters, and pandemic and epidemic diseases, human beings as a species have survived!

This chapter explores a number of healing modes, both ancient and modern. In addition, I include a historical overview on how such methods evolved, their purpose, and their practice. The relation of these healing practices to current religions is demonstrated primarily by listing the types of beliefs and practices found in a number of religions practiced in the United States. A description of various types of healers and remedies found and used in today's society concludes the chapter.

RELIGION AND HEALING

Religion plays a vital role in one's perception of health and illness. Just as culture and ethnicity are strong determinants in an individual's interpretation of the environment and the events within the environment, so, too, is religion. In fact, it is often difficult to distinguish between those aspects of a person's belief system that owe to religious background and those that stem from ethnic and cultural heritage. A given group of persons may share a common ethnicity and yet be of different religions; a group of people can share the same religion and yet have a variety of ethnic and cultural backgrounds. It is never safe to assume that all individuals of a given ethnic group practice or believe in the same religion. The point was embarrassingly driven home when I once asked a Chicano woman if she would like me to call the priest for her while her young son was awaiting a critical operation. The woman became angry with me. I could not understand why until I learned that she was a Methodist and not a Catholic. I had made an assumption, and I was wrong. She later told me that all Chicanos are not Catholic. After many years of having countless people make this same assumption, she had learned to react with anger.

Religion strongly affects the way people interpret and respond to the signs and symptoms of illness. Today, just as it did in antiquity, religion also plays a role in the rites surrounding both birth and death. So pervasive is religion that the diets of many people are determined by their religious beliefs. Religion and the religiosity of a given individual determine not only the role that his faith will play in the process of recovery, but in many instances precisely how he will respond to a given treatment and to the healing process. Each of these threads—religion, ethnicity, and culture—interweave into the fabric of each response of a particular person to treatment and healing.

Ancient Rituals

Many of the rituals that we observe at the time of birth and death have their origins in the practices of ancient human beings. Close your eyes for a few moments and picture yourself living thousands and thousands of years ago. There is no electricity, no running water, no bathroom, no plumbing. The nights are dark and cold. The only signs of the passage of time are the changing seasons and the apparent movement of the various planets and stars through the heavens. You are prey to all the elements, as well as to animals and the unknown. How do you survive? What sort of rituals and practices assist you in maintaining your equilibrium within this often hostile environment? It is from this milieu that many of today's practices sprang forth.

Generally speaking, there are three critical moments in the life of almost every human being: birth, marriage, and death.[2] One needs to examine the events and rites that were attendant on birth and death in the past and to demonstrate how many of them are not only relevant to our lives today but are also still practiced.

In the minds of early human beings, the number of evil spirits far exceeded the number of good spirits, and a great deal of energy and time was devoted to thwarting these spirits. They could be defeated by the use of gifts or rituals. Or, when the evil spirits had to be removed from a person's body, redemptive sacrifices were used. Once these evil spirits were expelled, they were prevented from returning by various magical ceremonies and rites. When a ceremony and incantation were found to be effective, they were passed on through the generations. It has been suggested and supported by scholars that, from this primitive beginning, organized religion came into being. Today, many of the early rites have survived in altered forms, and we continue to practice them.[3]

The power of the evil spirits was believed to endure for a certain length of time. The third, seventh, and fortieth days were the crucial days in the early life of the child and new mother; hence it was on these days, or the eighth day, that most of the rituals were observed. It was believed that during this period the newborn and the mother were at the greatest risk in the power of supernatural beings, and thus in a taboo state. "The concept underlying taboo is that all things created by or emanating from a supernatural being are his, or are at least in his power."[4] The person was freed from this taboo by certain rituals, depending on the practices of a given community. When the various rites were completed and the forty days were over, both the mother and child were believed to be redeemed from evil. The ceremonies that freed the person had a double character: they were partly magic and partly religious.

I have deliberately chosen to present the early practices of the Semitic peoples because their beliefs and practices evolved into the Judaic, Christian, and Islamic religions of today. Because the newborn baby and mother were considered to be vulnerable to the threats of evil spirits, many rituals were developed to protect them from these forces. For example, in some communities, the mother and child were separated from the rest of the community for a certain length of time, usually forty days. Various peoples performed precautionary measures such as rubbing the baby with different oils or garlic, swaddling the baby, and lighting candles.[5] In other communities, the baby and mother were closely watched for a certain length of time, usually seven days. (During this time span, they were believed to be intensely susceptible to the effects of evil—hence, close guarding was in order.) Orthodox Jews still refer to the seventh night of life as the "watchnight."[6]

The birth of a male child was considered to be more significant than that of a female, and countless rites were practiced in observance of this event. One form of ritual sacrifice was that of cutting off a lock of the child's hair, and then sprinkling his forehead with sheep's blood. This ritual was performed on the eighth day of life.[7] In other Semitic countries, when a child was named a sheep was sacrificed and asked to give protection to the infant. Depending on regional or tribal differences, the mother was or was not given parts of the sheep. It was believed that, if this sacrificial ritual was not performed on the seventh or eighth day of life, the child would die.[8] The sheep's skin was saved, dried, and placed in the child's bed for three or four years as protection from evil spirits.

Both the practice of cutting a lock of the child's hair and the sacrifice of an animal served as a ceremony of redemption. The child could also be redeemed from the taboo state by giving silver—the weight of which equaled the weight of the hair—to the poor.[9] Although not universally practiced, these rites are still observed, in one form or another, in some communities of the Arab world.[10]

Circumcision is closely related to the ceremony of cutting the child's hair and offering it as a sacrifice. Some authorities hold that the practice originated as a rite of puberty: a body mutilation performed to attract the opposite sex.[11] (Circumcision was practiced by many peoples throughout the ancient world; Alex Haley's *Roots* describes it as a part of initiating boys into manhood in Africa.) Other sources attribute it to the concept of the sanctity of the male organ and claim that it was derived from the practice of ancestor worship. The Jews of ancient Israel, as today, practiced circumcision on the eighth day of life.[12] The Moslems of Palestine circumcise their sons on the eighth day in the tradition that Mohammed established. In other Moslem countries, the ritual is performed anywhere from the tenth day to the seventh year of life.[13] Again, this sacrifice redeemed the child from being taboo in his early stages of life; once the sacrifice was made, the child entered the period of worldly existence. The rite of circumcision was accompanied by festivals of varying durations. Some cultures and kinship groups feasted for as long as a week.

The ceremony of baptism is also rooted in the past. It, too, symbolically expels the evil spirits, removes the taboo, and is redemptive. It is practiced mainly among members of the Christian faith, but the Yezidis and other non-Christian sects also perform the rite. Water was thought to possess magical powers and was used to cleanse the body from both physical and spiritual maladies, which included evil possession and other impurities. Usually, the child was baptized on the fortieth day of life. In some communities, however, the child was baptized on the eighth day. As alluded to earlier, the fortieth (or eighth) day was chosen because the ancients believed that—given performance of the particular ritual— this day marked the end of the evil spirits' influence. [14]

There were also a number of rituals that involved the new mother. For example, not only was she (along with her infant) removed from her household and community for forty days, but in many communities she had to practice ritual bathing before she could return to her husband, family, and community. Again, these practices were not universal and they varied in scope and intensity from people to people.

As to death, it was believed that the work of evil spirits and the duration of their evil—whether it was seven or forty days—surrounded the person, family, and community at the time. Rites evolved to protect both the dying and/or dead person and his remaining family from the evil spirits. The dying person was cared for in specific ways, such as ritual washing, and his grave was prepared in set ways—such as storing food and water for his journey. Further rituals were performed to protect the deceased's survivers from the harm believed to be rendered by the deceased's ghost: it was believed that this ghost could return from the grave and, if not carefully appeased, gravely harm his surviving relatives.[15]

Extensions to Today

Early human beings, in their quest for survival, strove to appease and prevent the evil spirits from interfering with their lives. Their beliefs seem simple and naive, yet the rituals that began in those years have evolved into those that still exist today. Attacks of the evil spirits were warded off with the use of amulets, charms, and the like. People recited prayers and incantations.[16] Because survival was predicated on people's ability to appease evil spirits, the prescribed rituals were performed with a great amount of care and respect. Undoubtedly, this accounts in part for the longevity of many of these practices through the ages. For example, circumcision and baptism still exist, even when the belief that they are being performed to release the child from a state of being taboo may not continue to be held. It is interesting also that adherence to a certain "time table" is maintained. For example, as stated, the Jewish religion mandates that the ritual of circumcision be performed on the eighth day of life.

The practice, too, of closely guarding the new mother and baby through the initial hours after birth is certainly not foreign to us. The mother is closely watched for hemorrhage and signs of infection; the infant initially is watched for signs of choking or respiratory distress. This form of observation is very intense. Could factors such as these have been what our ancestors watched for? If early human beings believed that evil spirits caused the frequent complications that surrounded the birth of a baby, then it stands to reason that they would seek to control or prevent these complications by adhering to astute observation, isolation, and rituals of redemption.

Table 3 is a useful summary of religious beliefs, with emphasis on how they may be expected to affect therapy.

BELIEFS THAT CAN AFFECT THERAPY

Ancient Forms of Healing

The crises of birth and death were certainly not the only ones to affect our ancestors. The earlier-described events of an illness also caused crises. Just as the people of ancient times developed ways

Table 3. Beliefs That Can Affect Therapy

1. Adventist

Seventh Day Adventist
Church of God
Advent Christian Church

Birth Opposed to infant baptism. Adults baptized by total immersion.

Death The dead are asleep until the return of Jesus Christ, at which time final rewards snd punishment will be given.

Health crisis Believe in man's choice and God's sovereignty. Taking of Communion or undergoing baptism may be desired. Some believe in divine healing and practice anointing with oil and use of prayer.

Diet No alcohol, coffee, or tea. The taking of all narcotics and stimulants is prohibited because the body is the temple of the Holy Spirit and should be protected. Many groups prohibit eating meat.

Beliefs Some sects regard Saturday as Sabbath. They accept the Bible literally, and keeping the commandments is the evidence of salvation. They believe their duty is to warn mankind to prepare for the second coming of Christ. Some oppose use of hypnotism in therapy.

2. American Indian

The approximately 300 different Indian tribal groups and geographically classified bands of Indians, each with their own culture, make it impossible to generalize about specific responses to specific situations. All have religion, magic, folklore, disease treatment, and herbal medicine; these differ from tribe to tribe. The medicine men, shamans, and conjurors in various tribes perform, by use of many different symbolic actions, against illnesses, social taboos, powers of nature, and "enemy-oriented" diseases. Protection against disease is sought by the help of superhuman powers. These practices have two distinct forms, according to the fundamental concept of the disease. Disease is conceived as taking two principal forms—one is the presence of a material object in the patient's body; the other is an effect of the absence of the soul from the body.

Many Indians today follow modern Christian religions, while some continue with their Indian beliefs.

Table 3. *(Continued)*

3. Armenian Church

Birth Baptism by total immersion 8 days after birth. Confirmation immediately following baptism.

Death Last rites practiced by the administration of Holy Communion.

Health crisis Taking Communion and "laying on of hands."

4. Baha'i

Birth No baptism.

Death No last rites.

Health crisis Prayer and, if medically permissible, fasting.

Diet Alcohol and drugs permitted only on doctor's prescription.

Beliefs No conflict between modern medicine and religion. The sick are specifically instructed in Baha'i scriptures to seek the advice of competent physicians. Spiritual health is felt to be conducive to physical health: Prayer adjunctive to healing by physical and chemical means is considered legitimate or even indispensable.

5. Baptist Bodies (27 bodies)

Birth Opposed to infant baptism. Only believers should be baptized, and it must be done by immersion.

Death Clergy seeks to minister by counsel and prayer with patient and family.

Health crisis Some Baptists believe and practice healing by the "laying on of hands."

Diet Some groups condemn coffee and tea.

Beliefs Supreme authority of Bible in all matters of faith and practice. Many Baptists condemn what the American Baptist Association terms "so-called modern science." Although the practical expression of this view is largely confined to opposition to Darwinism, resistance to medical therapy may be encountered. Most, however, believe that God works through the physician. Some who believe in predestination respond passively to care.

6. Brethren

Birth Baptism by immersion of those old enough to confess their faith.

Health crisis Anointment is practiced for physical healing and spiritual uplift.

Beliefs All members are ordained to ministry. Generally adhere to principle of conscientious objection to all wars.

Table 3. *(Continued)*

7. Buddhist Churches of America

Birth Rites such as infant presentation, affirmation, confirmation, or ordination are observed, but these are all held after the child has become mature enough to undergo these rites or for the mother to take the child with her.

Death Last rite chanting is often practiced at bedside soon after death. Contact the deceased's Buddhist priest or have the family make the contact.

Health crisis A Buddhist priest should be notified for counseling. However, it should be at the patient's or the family's request.

Beliefs They are in harmony with modern science. There is no divine punishment; every occurrence is dependent upon the law of causality and hence illness is due to karmic causes. This is a religion of supreme optimism as it teaches a way to overcome fears, anxieties, and apprehension. Special holy days are: January 1 and 16, February 15, March 21, April 8, May 21, July 15, September 1 and 23, December 8 and 31. Patients should be questioned how they feel about medical or surgical treatment on these days.

8. Black Muslim

Birth No baptism.

Death Carefully prescribed procedure for washing and shrouding the dead, and performing funeral rites.

Diet Prohibits alcoholic beverages, pork and meat of dead animals; also corn bread, collard greens, or other foods traditional among American blacks.

Beliefs General adherence to Moslem tenets is overlaid in many instances by antagonism to Caucasians, especially Christians and Jews. They do not indulge in activities such as sleeping more than is necessary to health and always maintain personal habits of cleanliness.

9. Church of Christ, Scientist (Christian Scientist)

Health crisis They deny the existence of health crises; sickness, sin, and death are errors of the human mind and can be destroyed by altering thoughts, not by drugs or medicines. They do not allow hypnotism or any form of psychotherapy which alters the "Divine Mind." A Christian Science Practitioner can be called to administer spiritual support; the *Christian Science Journal* contains a directory of Christian Science nurses available to help bandage wounds, set bones, etc.

Diet Alcohol, coffee, tobacco are seen as drugs, so not used.

Beliefs Disease is a human mental concept that can be dispelled by "spiritual truth." Many Christian Scientists adhere to this belief to the extent that they refuse all medical treatment, but each individual may decide whether

Table 3. *(Continued)*

he wishes to rely completely on Christian Science. Many adherents desire
the services of a Practitioner or Reader. The Church operates several nursing
homes that rely solely on such "spiritual" means of health maintenance.
They do not use drugs or blood transfusions, accept vaccines only when required by law, and do not seek biopsies or physical examinations.

10. Church of Christ (Temple Lot)

Birth No baptism until a minimum of 8 years, then baptism by immersion.
Death No last rites.
Health crisis Communion offered only to members of this church. Belief in
the anointing with oil and "laying on of hands" by the ministry for healing
of sick. Blood transfusions are acceptable and all normal medical practice.
Ministers (elders) will visit any who desire.
Beliefs No objection to "modern science" or therapy *per se*, but a simple
recognition of human limitations to wisdom and understanding. Sunday is
observed as the Sabbath but no objection to medical care on Sunday.

11. Church of God

Health crisis Adherents believe in divine healing through prayer, though more
liberal members do not prohibit medical therapy at the same time.
Beliefs "Speaking in tongues" is a sign of mystical experience.

12. Church of Jesus Christ of Latter Day Saints (Mormon)

Birth Baptism by immersion at 8 years or older.
Death Believe it proper to bury in ground; cremation is discouraged. Baptism
of the dead is held essential, though a living person may serve as proxy.
Preaching the Gospel to the dead is also practiced.
Health crisis Devout adherents believe in divine healing through the "laying
on of hands," though many do not prohibit medical therapy. The Church
maintains an extensive and well-funded welfare system, including financial
support for the sick.
Diet Prohibits alcoholic beverages, tobacco, hot drinks (tea, coffee), or any
other substance which may be injurious to the body. Encourages sparing
use of meats but prohibits none outright.
Beliefs There is a strong tradition of revelation through visions. A special
undergarment is often worn. Patients may desire to have a Church Priest-
hood holder administer the sacrament to them while in the hospital. This
would be on Sunday.

Table 3. *(Continued)*

13. Eastern Orthodox Churches

(Turkey, Egypt, Syria, Romania, Bulgaria, Cyprus, Albania, Poland, Czecho-
slovakia)

Birth Generally, these denominations believe in infant baptism by total immersion, followed immediately by confirmation.

Death Last rites obligatory if death is impending.

Health crisis Anointing of the sick is a form of healing by prayer.

Diet Restrictions dependent on particular sect.

14. Episcopalian

Birth Infant baptism is mandatory and especially urgent if prognosis is grave,
although aborted fetuses and stillborns are not baptized.

Death Last rites (Rite for the Anointing of the Sick) is not mandatory for all
members.

Health crisis Some believe in spiritual healing.

Diet Some abstain from meat on Fridays and some fast before receiving Holy
Communion, which may be daily.

Beliefs Many practice confession of sins and absolution.

15. Friends (Quakers)

Birth Do not baptize—at birth, an infant's name is recorded in official books.

Death Do not believe in life after this life.

Beliefs Are pacifists and conscientious objectors in wartime. Believe in plain
speech and dress and refusal of tithes, oaths. Believe God is in every man
and can be approached directly—religion inward, personal.

16. Greek Orthodox Church

Birth Baptism is significant. Prefer to baptize the child at least 40 days from
birth. If it is not possible to baptize by sprinkling or immersion, the
church allows the child to be baptized "in the air" by moving the child in
the form of the sign of the cross as appropriate words are said.

Death Last rites are the administration of the Sacrament of Holy Communion.
The priest should be called early enough so that the patient is still conscious.

Health crisis In most cases, each of these health-crisis situations must be
handled by an ordained priest, though a Deacon of the Church may also
serve in some cases. Usually a priest administers Holy Communion in the
hospital room in a procedure that takes only a few minutes. Some patients
may also want the Sacrament of Holy Unction, which the Priest can con-
duct in the hospital room in a brief time in an abbreviated service.

Table 3. *(Continued)*

Diet The Church usually prescribes a fast period, which means avoidance of meat and, in many cases, dairy products. These rules need not be enforced in cases of illness, especially when they may be of some harm to the health of the patient. Sometimes Orthodox patients will insist upon fasting even when in the hospital. If decision and desire to fast in the hospital do not interfere with medical procedures, there would be no reason for this to be refused. However, if this would adversely influence the medical condition of the patient, a priest should be called to convince the patient to forego fasting until his health is restored. The usual fasting days are Wednesday, Friday, and Lent.

17. Hindu

Death Certain prescribed rites are followed after death: The priest may tie thread around neck or wrist to signify blessing; the thread should not be removed. Immediately after death the priest will pour water into the mouth of the corpse; the family washes the body. They are particular about who touches their dead, and the bodies are cremated.

Diet There are many dietary restrictions that conform to individual sect doctrine. The patient should be questioned when admitted.

18. Islamic (Muslim/Moslem)

Birth The fetus before 130 days is treated as any other discarded tissue; after 130 days it must be treated as a fully developed human being.

Death The patient must confess sins and beg forgiveness before death, and the family should be present. The family washes, prepares, and places body facing Mecca. Only relatives or friends touch the body and unless required by law, there should be no postmortem; no body part should be removed.

Health crisis In pathologic conditions, faith healing is not acceptable unless the psychological condition of the patient is deteriorating. Then it is done for the patient's morale.

Diet All pork products are proscribed. Ninth month (Ramadan) daylight fasting is practiced.

Beliefs Older or more conservative Muslims often have a fatalist view that can militate against ready compliance with therapy.

19. Jehovah's Witnesses

Birth No infant baptism.

Death No last rites.

Health crises Adherents are generally absolutely opposed to blood transfusion, though individuals can sometimes be persuaded in emergencies. When par-

Table 3. *(Continued)*

ents refuse consent for a child's transfusion, it is often possible to obtain a
court order appointing some key hospital official temporary guardian of
the child. The official may then legally consent to the transfusion.

Beliefs The sect opposes the "false teachings" of other sects; opposition often
extends to modern science, including medicine. Some are pacifists and conscientious objectors in wartime; conversion of others is important. They
don't participate in nationalistic ceremonies or celebrate holidays by gift
giving.

20. Judaism

Birth Ritual circumcision is mandatory among Orthodox and Conservative
adherents on the 8th day. Reform Jews favor ritual circumcision, but not
as a religious imperative. A fetus is to be buried, not discarded.

Death Human remains are ritually washed following death by members of the
Ritual Burial Society, and the burial should take place as soon as possible.
Cremation is not in keeping with Jewish law. All Orthodox Jews and some
Conservatives are opposed to autopsy.

Diet Orthodox and Conservative Jews observe strict kosher dietary laws,
which mainly prohibit pork, shellfish, and the eating of meat with any
milk products. There are complex proscriptions and prescriptions regarding
food preparation. Reform Jews do not usually observe kosher dietary laws.

Beliefs Orthodox and Conservative adherents observe the Sabbath from sundown Friday to sundown Saturday. They may resist surgical procedures
during this period, unless a rabbi counsels that such procedures are medically necessary and are therefore permitted by Talmudic law. Amputated
limbs or organs or surgically removed body tissues should be available to
the family for burial. Parts of the body are not donated or removed, even
during autopsy.

21. Lutheran

Birth Baptize (only living) persons at 6-8 weeks following birth by pouring,
sprinkling, or immersing.

Death Last rites are optional.

Health crisis If the prognosis is grave, the patient may request the anointing
and blessing of the sick.

Beliefs Accept developments of science and technology but would raise ob-
jections if such techniques are administered unjustly or are clearly contrary
to Christian theology.

Table 3. *(Continued)*

22. Mennonite Church

Birth Baptism during early and middle teens.

Death No formal prescribed action. Personal assistance and prayer as appropriate while patient is still conscious.

Health crisis No taking of communion or laying on of hands.

Beliefs Not a sacramental church. There is a deep concern for the individual's dignity and self-determination, which would conflict with shock therapy or medicine or treatment affecting the individual's personality and will.

23. Methodist

Birth Baptism for children or adults.

Death Believe in divine judgment after death. Good will be rewarded and evil punished.

Health crisis Communion may be requested prior to surgery or similar crisis.

Beliefs Ministers counsel but do not hear confession. Donation of one's body or part of body at death is encouraged.

24. Moravian

Birth Infant baptism is usual, though they do not deny choice of adult baptism.

Death No last rites—when illness diagnosed as terminal, they do not believe that life should be extended at all costs; patient should be kept comfortable.

Health crisis Communion is received in both forms—both public and private communion. "Laying on of hands" for consecration of ordained persons—both male and female. No problem with blood transfusions or organ transplants.

Beliefs Disease is not a form of divine punishment, although they feel that breaking God's laws of "good stewardship" can often lead to physical problems. These, however, are not decreed by God.

25. Nazarene

Birth Baptism is parent's option, not considered a saving sacrament. No need for a baby, including a fetus, or an adult who is dying to be baptized.

Death No last rites—cremation is permitted, term stillborn infants are buried.

Health crisis Local pastor will administer communion and laying on of hands, which are means of grace. Adherents believe in divine healing, but not exclusive of medical treatment.

Diet Use of alcohol and tobacco prohibited.

Beliefs No conflicts with modern science.

Table 3. *(Continued)*

26. Pentecostal (Assembly of God, Four-square Church)

Birth Water baptism by complete single immersion after age of accountability.
Death No last rites.
Health crisis No inhibitions against blood transfusions or medical care.
Believe in possibility of divine healing through prayer. Anointing with oil
may be practiced with laying on of hands.
Diet Abstain from alcohol, tobacco, eating blood and strangled animals.
Individual may resist pork.
Beliefs Some insist illness is divine punishment but most consider illness an
intrusion of Satan. Deliverance from sin and sickness are provided for in
atonement. Pray for divine intervention in health matters and seek to reach
God in prayer for themselves and others when ill.

27. Orthodox Presbyterian

Birth Sprinkling most common in infant baptism.
Death Last rites not a sacramental procedure; they read Scripture and pray.
Health crisis Communion administered when appropriate and convenient;
blood transfusion acceptable when advisable; no formal laying on of hands
ceremony; prayer appropriate; local pastor or elder should be called.
Belief True science to be utilized for relief of suffering and recognized as a
gift of the Creator. Full forgiveness through genuine repentance for any
illness connected with a sin. Think of heaven and hell in material terms.

28. First Church of Religious Science

Birth No baptism.
Death No last rites.
Health crisis No communion or laying on of hands— believe only in prayer.
Beliefs No objection to medical science. Do not believe in divine punishment,
only absolute goodness of God.

29. Roman Catholic

Birth Infant baptism is mandatory and especially urgent if prognosis is grave.
Baptism is demanded if an aborted fetus may not be clinically dead. For
baptismal purposes, "death" is a certainty only if there is obvious evidence
of tissue necrosis.
Death The Rite for the Anointing of the Sick is mandatory. If the prognosis
is grave, the patient or the family may request it.

Table 3. *(Continued)*

Health crisis The patient or family may desire that a major amputated limb be buried in consecrated ground. There is no blanket mandate for this, but it may be required within a given diocese.

Diet Most hospital patients are exempt from fasting or abstaining from meat on Ash Wednesday and Good Friday. Some older Catholics may still adhere to the former rule of abstaining from meat on all Fridays.

30. Russian Orthodox

Birth Baptism by priest only. Immersion three times as John the Baptist did and only on certain days.

Death Do not believe in autopsies, embalming, or cremation. At death arms are crossed and fingers set in a cross. Clothing at death must be of natural fiber so that the body will change to ashes sooner.

Health crisis Cross necklace is important and should be replaced immediately when patient returns from surgery.

Diet During Lent, Wednesdays, and Fridays, they don't eat meat or dairy products.

Beliefs Important not to shave male patients, exception only for surgery.

31. Spiritualism

Diet Many maintain a vegetarian diet.

Beliefs Generally accept the main ideas of Christianity plus the belief in the continuation of personal identity after death, termed a "change." Communication with the dead is thought possible. Family members may therefore devote much time and energy to an attempt, often believed successful, to communicate with a dead relative.

32. Unitarian/Universalist

Birth Some practice infant baptism; most consider it unnecessary.

Death Attitudes toward immortality vary widely. Cremation preferred to burial.

Health crisis No official sacraments. Reason and practicality are most important.

Beliefs Believe each individual has right to approach values in own way. Believe God helps those who help themselves. At times, some may prefer not to have clergy visit them in hospital since they assume responsibility themselves. Emphasize use of reason and knowledge and the use of the best of modern knowledge in relation to religion.

of dealing with the events that surrounded birth and death, they evolved elaborate systems of healing. The cause of an illness, once again, was attributed to the forces of evil, which originated either within or outside of the body. Thus early forms of healing dealt with the removal of evil. Once a method of treatment was found effective, it was passed down through the generations in slightly altered forms.

The people who healed were often those who received the gift of healing from a "divine" source. They frequently received this gift in a vision, and were unable to explain to others how they knew what to do. Other healers learned their skills from their parents. Most of the healers with acquired skills were women, who subsequently passed their knowledge on to their daughters. People who used herbs and other preparations to remove the evil from the sick person's body were known as herbalists. Other healers included bone setters and the midwives, and although early humankind did not separate ills of the body from ills of the mind, there were healers who were more adept at solving the problems of the individual by using early forms of "psychotherapy."

The use of natural products—such as wild herbs and berries that were accessible to the healers—developed into today's science of pharmacology. Early humankind had a wealth of knowledge with respect to the medicinal properties of the plants, trees, and mushrooms in their environment. They knew how to prepare certain concoctions from the barks and roots of trees, and others from berries and wild flowers. As an example, purple foxglove was the "digitalis" of yesteryear: it slowed the heart rate.

If the source of sickness-causing evil was within the body, treatment involved drawing the evil out of the body. This may have been accomplished through the use of purgatives that caused either vomiting or diarrhea, or by blood-letting: "bleeding" the patient or "sucking out" blood. (The barbers of medieval Europe did not originate this practice; bleeding was done in ancient times.) Leeching was another method used to remove corrupt humors from the body, and the reader may recall from Chapter 3 that it was mentioned by a student whose grandmother had treated illness by that method.

If the source of the evil was outside of the body, there were a

number of ways to deal with it. One source of "external" evil
was witchcraft. In a given community, there were often many
people (or a single person) who were "different" from the other
people. Quite often, when an unexplainable or untreatable illness
occurred, it was these people (or person) who were seen as the
causative agents. In such a belief-system it follows logically that
successful treatment of such a problem depended on the identification and punishment of the individuals (or person) who were
believed responsible for the disease. (Certainly, the practice of
scapegoating is in part derived from this belief.) By removing
the guilty people (or person) from the community, or by punish-
ing them, the disease would be cured. In some communities, the
healers themselves were seen as witches and the possessors of evil
skills. How easy it was for ancient humankind to turn things
around and blame the person with the skills to treat the disease
for causing the disease!

Numerous rituals were involved in the treatment of ill people.
Often the sick person was isolated from the rest of the family
and community. In addition, it was customary to chant special
prayers and incantations on his behalf; sacrifices and dances were
often performed in an effort to cure his ills. Often the rituals of
the healer involved reciting incantations in a language foreign to
the ears of the general population ("speaking in tongues") and
the use of practices that were strange and alien to the observers.
Small wonder, then, as superstition abounded, that at times the
healers themselves were ostracized by the population.

Another cause of illness was believed to be the *envy* of people
within the community. Consequently, as we mentioned in an
earlier chapter, the best method of preventing such illness was
to avoid provoking the envy of one's friends and neighbors. The
treatment was to do away with whatever was provoking the envy—
even though the act may in many ways have prevented a person
from accomplishing his "mission in life," and the fear of being
"responsible" may have been psychologically damaging.

Today we tend to view the healing methods of ancient people
as being primitive. Yet to fully appreciate their efficacy, we need
only make the simple observation that these methods in many
forms exist today and have aided the survival of humankind!

Healing Today

It is not an accident or coincidence that today, more so than in recent years, we are not only curious but vitally concerned about the ways of healing that our ancestors employed. There are those who choose to condemn the health system, with more vociferous critics such as Illich citing its failure to create a utopia for humankind.[17] It is obvious to those who embrace a more moderate viewpoint that diseases continue to occur and that they outflank our ability to cure or prevent them. Once again, many people are electing to seek out the services of people who are knowledgeable in the arts of healing and folk medicine. Many patients may elect, at some point in their lives, and more specifically during an illness, to use modalities outside the medical establishment. Thus it is important to understand these treatment methods and have some working knowledge of them.

For example, the current popularity of "health foods" has given rise to the popular use of various diets to prevent illness. In addition, health-food stores make available a number of medicinal teas and herbs. (A listing of commonly used herbs is presented in Table 4.) There are almost one hundred herbal teas listed in a small paperback entitled *Herbal Tea Book*.[18] The herbs are alphabetically listed, and the source and use of each are given. There is an even larger listing in the book *Herbs: Medicine and Mysticism*[19] by Sybil Leek, who is known as one of the "world's foremost astrologers and witches." This book has a wide reading audience.

As also discussed in an earlier chapter, Laetrile is considered by some to be a cure for cancer. Apart from numerous political ramifications within the health-care system, Laetrile creates another dilemma. If it has healing powers--even if limited to making people feel a little better until they die—then one can appreciate its usefulness.[20] But if Laetrile does not live up to what its proponents claim it is able to do, then the public is falling prey to a pseudomedical hoax.

It is difficult to sort out which aspects of folk medicine have merit and which are a hoax. From the viewpoint of the consumer—if he has faith in the efficacy of an herb, a diet, a pill, and/or a healer—it is not a hoax. From the viewpoint of the medical establishment, jealous of its territorial claim, this same herb, diet, pill, or healer is indeed a hoax if it is *ineffective* and

Table 4. Commonly Used Herbs

Herb	Action	Use	Administration
Alfalfa (or Lucerne)	Stimulant; nutritive	Arthritis; weight gain; strength-giving	1 oz. herb to 1 pint water; drink 1 cupful as tea
Anise (seed used)	Stimulant; aromatic; relaxant	Flatulence; dry coughs	2 tsp. of seed to ½ pint water; dose—1-3 tsp. often
Bayberry (bark used)	Astringent; stimulant; emetic	Sore-throat gargle; cleanses stomach; douche; rinse for bleeding gums	1 oz. powdered bark to 1 pint water; drink as tea
Blessed thistle	Diaphoretic; stimulant; emetic	Reduces fevers; breaks up colds; digestive problems	1 oz. herb to 1 pint water; small doses as desired
Bugleweed	Aromatic; sedative; tranquilizer; astringent	Coughs; relieves pulmonary bleeding; increases appetite	1 oz. herb to 1 pint water; drink by glassful often
Catnip (leaves)	Diaphoretic; tonic; antispasmodic	Helpful in convulsions; produces perspiration	1 oz. leaves to 1 pint water (measured by teaspoonsful); tsp.
Cayenne pepper (fruit and seed)	Stimulant; toxic	Purest and most positive stimulant in herbal medicine; healing of burns and other wounds; relieves toothaches	Powder in small doses; by mouth or topical
Chestnut, Horse (bark and fruit)	Astringent; narcotic; tonic	Bark used for fevers; fruit to treat rheumatism	Bark: 1 oz. to 1 pint water, tsp. 4 times per day; fruit: tincture 10 drops twice per day

(Continued)

Table 4. *(Continued)*

Herb	Action	Use	Administration
Chicory (root)	Diuretic; laxative	Liver enlargement; gout; rheumatic complaints	1 oz. root to 1 pint water; take freely
Corn silk	Diuretic; mild stimulant	Irritated bladder; urinary stones; trouble with prostate bland	2 oz. in 1 pint water; take freely
Dandelion (root)	Diuretic; tonic	Used in many patent medicines; general body stimulant; used chiefly with kidney and liver disorders	Roasted roots are ground and used like coffee; small cup once or twice per day
Ergot (fungus)	Uterine stimulant; sedative; hemostatic	Menstrual disorders; stops hemorrhage	Liquid extract 10-20 minims by mouth
Eucalyptus	Antiseptic; antispasmodic; stimulant	Inhale for sore throat; apply to ulcers and other wounds	Local application or fluid extract in small doses by mouth
Fennel (seeds)	Aromatic; carminative (expels air from bowels)	Gas; gout; colic in infants; increases milk in nursing mothers	Pour water (½ pint) on 1 tsp. of seeds; take freely
Garlic (juice)	Diaphoretic; diuretic; stimulant; expectorant	Treats colds; diuretic; antiseptic	Juice, 10-30 drops
Goldenrod (leaves)	Aromatic; stimulant	Sore throat; general pain; colds; rheumatism	1 oz. leaves to 1 pint water; small dose often
Hollyhock (flowers)	Diuretic	Chest complaints	1 oz. flowers to 1 pint water; drink as much as needed

Ivy (leaves)	Cathartic; diaphoretic	Poultices on ulcers and abscesses	As a poultice
Ivy, poison (leaves)	Irritant; stimulant; narcotic	Rheumatism; sedative for the nervous system	Liquid extract 5-30 drops
Juniper berries	Diuretic; stimulant	Bladder and kidney problems; gargles; digestive aid	Oil of berries 1-5 drops
Licorice (root)	Demulcent	Coughs; prevents thirst	Powdered root
Lily of the valley (flower)	Cardiac; diuretic; stimulant	Headaches	½ oz. of flowers to 1 pint water; tbsp. doses
Marigold (flowers and leaves)	Diaphoretic; stimulant	Flowers and leaves made into a salve for skin eruptions; relieves sore muscles; amenorrhea	1 oz. herbs and petals to 1 pint water; tbsp. on mouth or topical application
Mistletoe (leaves)	Nervine; antispasmodic; tonic; narcotic	Epilepsy and hysteria; painful menstruation; induces sleep	2 oz. to ½ pint water; 1 tbs. often
Mustard (leaves)	Cooling; sedative	Hoarseness (excellent aid in recovering the voice)	Liquid extract; small doses
Nightshade, deadly (poison) (leaves and root)	Narcotic; diuretic; sedative; antispasmodic	Eye diseases; increases urine; stimulates circulation	Powdered leaves and root; small amounts

(Continued)

Table 4. *(Continued)*

Herb	Action	Use	Administration
Papaya leaves	Digestive	Digestive disorders; fresh leaves: dry wounds	Papain; small doses
Rosemary (leaves) (herb)	Astringent; diaphoretic; tonic; stimulant	Prevents baldness; cold; colic; nerves; strengthens eyes	1 oz. herb to 1 pint water; small doses
Saffron (flower pestils)	Carminative; diaphoretic	Amenorrhea; dysmenorrhea; hysteria	1 drachm flower pestils in 1 pint water; teacup doses
Thyme (dried herb)	Antiseptic; antispasmodic; tonic	Perspiration; colds; coughs; cramps	1 oz. herb to 1 pint water; tbs. doses often

Source: Sybil Leek, *Herbs: Medicine and Mysticism* (Chicago: Henry Regnery, 1975), pp. 73-235.

prevents the person from using the method of treatment that the physician-healer believes is effective.

There are numerous healers in the general population, some of whom are legitimate and some of whom are not. They range from housewives and priests to gypsies and "witches." Countless people seek their services. I have had occasion to meet with several of these folk healers. Without attempting to make a value judgment, I will merely report on their skills and methods.

One healer has an office in a community near to where I live. He charges a nominal fee for consultation with either groups or individuals and then gives advice on how to solve a problem. He does not see physically ill people but prefers to help people who have moderate emotional and practical problems. His primary objective is to help people solve these problems. This man tends to be quite popular with young adults in the area, as he lends a "willing ear" and is "not too expensive." He does not keep his clients waiting long, and often the brief wait proves to be interesting because the waiting room is always the scene of an open discussion about his talents.

Another healer I knew was a young college student. He believed that he possessed certain spirits and skills that enabled him to heal. He had visions that interpreted for him the problems and ills of his clients. This young man maintained a special altar in his room, where he prayed to the "spirits." At that time, he did not charge for his services because he had just received the "message," and the art of healing was new to his experiences. He admitted that he had formerly been a drug addict, but was now enrolled in college and hoped to use his education and healing skills to make life better for the people of the streets.

The third healer I am personally acquaintainted with is a practicing Catholic priest; he is extremely reluctant to call himself a "healer." Yet he does claim to have witnessed and participated in numerous healings. He conducts prayer meetings in his parish. He comes to my classes and lectures to the students on healing and the Charismatic movement within the Catholic Church.[21] He defines healing as the "satisfactory response to crises by a group of people, individually or corporately." "Healing," as he explains it, "is applied in a broad, holistic approach; that is, body, mind, and spirit are not separated." His vision of reality is that of a man being full with the spirit of God. According to this priest, the healer has the ability to *heal* but not really to *cure*. He further explains that there are "three types of illness: spiritual, physical, and mental." In this context, faith is the underlying basis of healing, although he questions whether faith is the only component. Healing becomes a living process whereby that which is wounded or broken becomes whole.

A review of healing and spiritual literature reveals that there are four types of healing.

Spiritual Healing

This is used when a person is experiencing an illness of the spirit. The cause of suffering is personal sin. The treatment modality is repentence, which is followed by a natural healing process.

Inner Healing

This is used when a person is suffering from an emotional (mental) illness. The root of the problem may lie in the person's conscious or unconscious mind. The treatment method is to heal the person's memory. The healing process is delicate and sensitive, and exposure takes considerable time and effort.

Physical Healing

This is used when a person is suffering from a disease or has been involved in an accident that resulted in some form of bodily damage. Laying on of hands and/or speaking in tongues usually accompanies physical healing. The person is prayed over by both the "leader" and members of a prayer group.

The priest referred to above related an incident in which one of the members of the group was experiencing difficulty with ulcers and was not responding to conventional medical treatment. The man, who initially was embarrassed by the idea, allowed the prayer group and the priest to pray over him. In a short time, to his surprise, he recovered from his ulcers.

Deliverance or Exorcism

This is used when the body and mind are the victim of evil from the outside. In order to effect treatment, the person must be delivered or exorcised from the evil. The continuing popularity of films such as *The Exorcist* gives testimony to the return of these types of beliefs. Incidentally, the priest who has lectured in my classes stated that he does not, as yet, lend credence to exorcisms, however, he was guarded enough not to discount it either.

Further Comments

Another form of treatment is "auric healing." John Richard Turner of Waltham, Massachusetts, explains that "from the moment of birth until the last breath is taken, a person has a bioenergetic field surrounding his body." This field of energy is known as an "aura." If strong enough, it is believed to be transmittable and to have healing powers. By the use of touch, the person with the auric powers is able to effect cure for an ill person.[22] Mr. Turner, who is fairly well known in the Boston area, also claims to be quite popular in California. He states that he visits patients in the hospital along with the physician and that he has been quite successful in treating people in that setting.

There is also a film available that demonstrates how some individuals relate to folk healers. The film, "We Believe in Nino Fidencio," is a documentary on folk curing and penitent pilgrimages in northern Mexico. Shot in October 1971 in northern Mexico by Dr. and Mrs. Jon Olson (who were in Mexico doing field research), the film is concerned with:

> ... the belief system and ceremonies surrounding a folk curer, Fidencio Constantino, who practiced in Nuevo Leon from the early 1920's until his death in 1938, and who is presently the central figure in a widespread curing cult. Twice each year, upon the anniversaries of his birth and death, Espinazo (a town of about 300 population) is inundated by 10,000 to 15,000 people from Mexico and the United States who make pilgrimages in hopes of a cure and/or help from the Nino. It was during one of these celebrations that the film was made.
>
> Believers combine elements of traditional Catholicism, Indian dances, herbology, and laying-on-of-hands in effecting cures. It is believed that certain individuals receive the Nino's power to heal. They are called "Cajitas" or "Materias" (women), and "Cajones" (men)—"receptacles" of the Nino's power—and they cure in the name of Nino Fidencio and God. During the celebrations they roam Espinazo curing all who

wish a cure-blessing. There are several "holy places" in Espinazo where curing is conducted: Fidencio's tomb, "temple," and death bed, two trees, a cemetary hill, the hill of the bell, and the "charco" or mudpond, where Fidencio conducted baptisms to cure his patients.

The film includes references to other curing alternatives, and attempts to present some of the reasons why the believers continue to select this curing method in the face of modern medical alternatives in nearby towns and cities.

As previously stated, Dr. Olson first learned about this cult in 1968-1969 while doing field research in Mina, a community in the same county as Espinazo. It was during this time that the Olsons met members of the cult (in Mina and Espinazo) including the local "materia," Cayetana, who appear in the film. The narration of the film is based on information and acutal recorded interviews given by participants in the cult. Jon Olson is presently an Assistant Professor of Anthropology at California State University at Los Angeles.

Extensive study of the Nino Fidencio complex has been done by Professor June Macklin (Connecticut College).[23]

CONCLUSIONS

I hasten to reiterate that this chapter is no more than an *overview* of the topics introduced; the amount of relevant knowledge could fill many books. The issues raised here are those that, I think, have special meaning to the practice of nursing, medicine, and health-care delivery. We must be aware (1) of what people may be thinking that may differ from our own thoughts and (2) that sources of *help* exist outside the traditional medical community. As the beliefs of ethnic communities of color are explored in later chapters, I shall attempt to delineate who are specifically recognized and used as healers by the members of the community, and I shall describe some of the forms of treatment employed by each community.

REFERENCES

1. Joyce Leeson, "Paths to Medical Care in Lasaka, Zambia," (unpublished thesis, University of Manchester, England; preliminary findings, 12 July, 1967) p. 14.

2. Julian Morgenstern, *Rites of Birth, Marriage, Death and Kindred Occasions among the Semites* (Chicago: Quadrangle Books, 1966) p. 3.
3. Ibid., p. 5.
4. Ibid., p. 31.
5. Ibid., pp. 22-30.
6. Ibid., pp. 22-30.
7. Ibid., p. 36.
8. Ibid., p. 87.
9. Ibid., p. 46.
10. Ibid., p. 47.
11. Ibid., p. 48.
12. Ibid., p. 58.
13. Ibid., p. 53.
14. Ibid., p. 82.
15. Ibid., p. 117-160.
16. Ibid., p. 186.
17. Ivan Illich, *Medical Nemesis: The Expropriation of Health* (London: Marion Bogars, 1975).
18. Ann Adrian and Judith Dennis, *Herbal Tea Book* (San Francisco: Health Publishing Co., 1976).
19. Sybil Leek, *Herbs: Medicine and Mysticism* (Chicago: Henry Regnery, 1975).
20. John A. Richardson and Patricia Griffin, *Laetrile Case Histories* (New York: Bantam, 1977).
21. Francis MacNutt, *Healing* (Notre Dame, Ind.: Ave Maria Press, 1974); Morton T. Kelsey, *Healing and Christianity* (New York: Harper, 1973).
22. John Richard Turner, notes from a lecture delivered at a meeting of the World's Future Society held at Boston College, 16 March, 1977.
23. Flyer on the film "We Believe in Nino Fidencio" (Jon and Natalie Olson, P.O. Box 14914, Long Beach, Calif. 90814).

BIBLIOGRAPHY: HEALING

Belgum, David, editor. *Religion and Medicine.* Ames: Iowa State University Press, 1967.

> This book explores two dimensions of healing: religion and medicine. The essays it contains explore the nature of humankind and its problems in sickness and health.

Kelsey, Morton T. *Healing and Christianity.* New York: Harper, 1973.

> Kelsey presents a comprehensive history of the sacrament of healing in the Christian Church from Biblical times to the present.

Leek, Sybil. *Herbs: Medicine and Mysticism.* Chicago: Henry Regnery, 1975.

> Multiple herbs and their uses are described—both those in current use among the general population and those used among the Hopi Indian tribes.

MacNutt, Francis. *Healing.* Notre Dame, Ind.: Ave Maria Press, 1974.

> This book explores the Charismatic movement in the Catholic Church. It describes in great detail the multiple forms of healing within the Church.

_____. *The Power to Heal.* Notre Dame, Inc.: Ave Maria Press, 1977.

> In this book, Father MacNutt further describes his experiences within the healing ministry. He addresses such topics as "Healing Through Touch," "Soaking Prayer," "Suffering and Death," and "When and When Not to Pray."

Montgomery, Ruth, *Born to Heal.* New York: Coward, McCann, 1973.

> This is the story of a dynamic man and his seemingly miraculous cures of tragic ailments, which run the gamut of human suffering. Mr. A. first devoted himself to healing in 1941 and experienced conflict with the traditional health system.

Morgenstern, Julian. *Rites of Birth, Marriage, Death, and Kindred Occasions among the Semites.* Chicago: Quadrangle Books, 1966.

> Morgenstern presents a fascinating history of the rites that preceded today's religions. It is hard to follow, because the author tends to jump back and forth, but it is well worth the effort because its content is quite interesting.

Scott, W. Richard, and Volkhart, Edmund H. *Medical Care Readings in the Sociology of Medical Institutions.* New York: Wiley, 1966.

> This anthology explores such topics as the varieties of healers, the relationships between healers and patients, and relationships between patients and hospitals.

FURTHER SUGGESTED READINGS

Books

Adrian, Ann, and Dennis, Judith. *Herbal Tea Book.* San Fransisco: Health Publishing Co., 1976.

Cassell, Eric J. *The Healer's Art: A New Approach to the Doctor-Patient Relationship.* Philadelphia: Lippincott, 1976.

Kiev, Ari, editor. *Magic, Faith, and Healing: Studies in Primitive Psychiatry Today.* New York: Free Press of Glencoe, 1969.

Krippner, Stanley, and Villoldo, Alberto. *The Realms of Healing.* Millbrae, California: Celestial Arts, 1976.

Ortez y Pino, Jose, III. *The Herbs of Galisteo and Their Powers.* Santa Fe, N.M.: Vergara, 1972.
Sweet, Muriel, *Common Edible and Useful Plants of the West.* Healdsbury, California: Naturegraph, 1962.

Articles

Grad, Bernard. "Some Biological Effects of the 'Laying on of Hands:' A Review of Experiments with Animals and Plants." *Journal of the American Society for Psychical Research* 59(1965): 94-127.
Kleinman, Arthur M. "Some Issues for a Comparative Study of Medical Healing." *International Journal of Social Psychiatry* 19 (1973): 159-165.
Krieger, Dolores. "Therapeutic Touch: The Imprimatur of Nursing." *American Journal of Nursing* 75 (1975): 784-787.
Leeson, Joyce. "Paths to Medical Care in Lusaka, Zambia." Unpublished thesis, University of Manchester, England; preliminary findings, 12 July, 1967.

UNIT III
A Barrier and a Bridge

This unit explores two pervasive issues: poverty as a barrier to health care and whether health care is a "right." A question posed is whether people continue to use traditional methods of healing because they *believe* in them or because they are denied access to fee-for-service medical care.

CHAPTER 7

Poverty:
The Barrier
to Health Care

Manuel Spector

Numerous barriers prevent people from seeking health care, utilizing health resources, and complying with both preventive and therapeutic regimens. These barriers include language difficulties, unavailability of health-care resources, inaccessibility of health-care resources, and a personal, individual inability to "understand" and relate to the deliverers of health care. However, the outstanding barrier by far to health care is *poverty*. Not only does poverty render the person less able to seek health care but it also accounts for the greater probability of the "poor" person's acquiring an illness.

What is poverty? To recite figures, list incomes, or enumerate problems answers the question only in part. Poverty "is a relative term that reflects a judgment made on the basis of standards prevailing in the community. The standards change in time and place; what is judged poverty in one community might be regarded as wealth in another."[1]

Is there poverty in the United States, the wealthiest nation on earth? YES. A recent study reported in the *New York Times* found that "poverty is far less persistent but much more pervasive in American life than most would have thought."[2]

In part, poverty is the result of the unequal distribution of means and privileges. This means that from all that is available—in assets, goods, and services—some people have too much, others too little. The apparent discrepancies are uncovered when one sees what his neighbor has. In this country of "plenty" the person with an income of $5,000 sees himself as poor. In a "developing" or "underdeveloped" country where the standard incomes are much lower, the same $5,000 puts a person in a much higher socio-economic class. The latest United States statistical reports hold that an annual income of less than $10,000 is marginal for a family of four. The poverty line rests far below that figure.

It is a part of the reality of life that we judge people by what they have and what they know. Therefore, a poor, uneducated or undereducated person is not held in high esteem or granted as much respect as his more wealthy, well-educated, well-dressed counterpart. Some individuals and communities view poverty as the result of evil: the poor experience deserved divine punishment for their "evil" or "lazy" ways. Others see poverty as a blight that is visited upon man by a divine force so that others will learn to appreciate what they have. Yet others regard poverty as an opportunity to meet their own religious obligations by "helping their poor brothers."

In some societies poverty is taken for granted and ignored. This was the case in the United States in the past; to many it is still the case today. When the term *poverty* is mentioned in more affluent communities, it is generally associated with the term *needy*, which conjures up the need to assist the poor. A working definition of *poverty* in terms of values is as follows: a condition of being in want of something that is needed, desired, or generally recognized as having some value. Poverty can also be a cultural phenomenon. Poverty, starvation, and death caused by lack of resources or exposure are seen as absolute forms of poverty. In all cases poverty is relative. Poverty is a condition the essence of which is inequality.

Often poverty is both visible and invisible. Visible poverty can be a lack of material and resources, inadequate housing, inferior clothing, etc. Invisible poverty is marked by social and cultural deprivation.

Many Americans take poverty for granted. Americans generally accept the term "pockets of poverty," and acknowledge the existence of this phenomenon in most urban areas and in many rural areas. Essentially the phrase has come to connote limited employment opportunities, inferior educational opportunities, lack of or inferior medical services and health-care facilities, poor sanitation, deteriorating housing, and an absence of public services. The very opposite situations are by and large taken for granted by most middle-class families.

Invisible poverty is a growing social problem in our society, and shows no sign of abatement. It affects the elderly and the recently retired, those with fixed incomes, the working poor, and those who are not able to purchase health-care insurance and cannot afford to pay for health care. The working poor have high enough incomes to be considered ineligible for governmental health-care programs.

The chief cause of this invisible poverty lies in the inflationary economic condition of the country and the world. Inflation diminishes purchasing power, thereby making common human needs—such as food, shelter, housing, and health care—almost inaccessible for most familes in the lower socioeconomic brackets. Governmental mechanisms for assisting those in need—such as social security, unemployment insurance, supplemental income assistance, and food stamps—are seldom adequate to meet basic family needs. Such programs are now even less adequate in helping the poor to keep up with economic pressures brought on by escalating costs in our free-market economy.

POVERTY REDISCOVERED

The complacency that permeated America during the post-World War II years included the widely held belief among most middle- and upper-income classes that hard-core poverty had been eliminated or brought under control. In 1958, John Kenneth Galbraith in his brilliant book, *The Affluent Society,* illuminated the problem of poverty as affecting minorities, migratory workers, the populations of the Appalachian, Ozark, and Piedmont regions, and most of the rural South. Galbraith referred to this destitution as "insular poverty" related to low income and insufficient wages.[3] In addition, he found that millions of persons were living in poverty because of poor health, crippling diseases, education and training that were either lacking or inferior, alcoholism, drug addiction, large family size, unemployment or underemployment, and racial or ethnic discrimination. This type of poverty Galbraith referred to as "case poverty." Still, in the midst of unparalled economic growth and prosperity, it was difficult to imagine the existence of various levels of poverty in our society.

In 1963, another significant study of poverty by Michael Harrington[4] lucidly showed how poverty in the United States had reached epidemic proportions, with about 36 million people— or 1 out of 5—having an income below the poverty line. Here, in the richest country on earth, there was indeed poverty! While many of the economic-assistance and social-insurance programs had some effect, much chronic poverty remained. By 1975, about 30 million Americans were still classified as having an income that was below the poverty line; 12 percent of the population had an income of under $5,500 for a family of four.[5] Large clusters of people—especially minorities, the elderly, rural residents, and migrants—remained closed off from the apparent benefits of the economic prosperity of the 1950s and 1960s.

In the 1970s, the most prominent factors effecting change in the economic status of the United States were those that affected family composition: such as divorce and new children's being added to the re-formed family, and loss of purchasing power because of inflation. According to a University of Michigan study "there is virtually no evidence that personal attitudes such as self-confidence, ambition, and motivation (typical middle class values deemed as desirable for all Americans, especially the poor) have much to do with economic improvement."[6] In fact, the various public-welfare programs run by the Federal and state governments at an annual cost of more that $30 billion are, surprisingly, "relatively unimportant components of change in family well-being."[7] The study further states that persistently poor people are likely to live in households headed by a person who is 65 years old; who is Black, female, or disabled; and who has little formal education.[8] Therefore, it is clear that those among us who are impoverished will continue to be impoverished and will continue to defy efforts to eliminate their indigence. Thus poverty and its many causes must be regarded as the end result of many forces, factors, and historic roots. For this reason poverty can be analyzed from three distinct perspectives: geographic, social, and psychologic.

Three Perspectives

"Geographic" poverty is seen in the numerous pockets of poverty in the United States: in most dense urban areas (usually localized in the ghettos) and in nonurbanized regions such as Appalachia, the Deep South, Lower Southwest, and northern New England. In fact, some experts suggest that rural America is the seat of hard-core and long-lasting poverty.

Factors that enter into geographic poverty include the combination of social and economic conditions that have failed to create legitimate economic and work opportunities. Where such poverty exists, local conditions perpetuate the unequal distribution of public services in education, health, sanitation, employment, transportation, welfare, and political reforms. After many efforts to reform and improve this pattern of geographic poverty, it has become evident that without massive outside assistance local government cannot eradicate these endemic socioeconomic conditions. Once born into a situation of extreme want in a region of poverty, one is likely to be condemned to this level of indigence or destitution unless he moves elsewhere. This situation occurs because social mobility, education, job training, and employment opportunities are not promoted in these settings.

"Social" factors of poverty refer to demographic characteristics such as race, age, sex, education, family size, income, and work, all of which determine the social position a person occupies in a particular society. Social scientists state that the most obvious distinguishing characteristics of poverty are race and age. In terms of visible poverty, Blacks, Hispanics, Native Americans (Indians), and the elderly are substantially orverrepresented in the ranks of the impoverished in America. In 1971 Blacks accounted for 29 percent of the poverty population but only 11 percent of the national population.[9] Similar statistics are given for Hispanics. Whites account for only 9 percent of the nation's poor. Obviously all persons are *not* created equal.

Age is another distinguishing factor in poverty. The incidence of poverty among those who are 65 years of age or older is growing as inflation greedily consumes whole chunks of incomes. Retirement, whether voluntary or compulsory, has a direct link to the economic status of the elderly. On the other end of the age spectrum, youth and children are more likely to be overrepresented in the ranks of the poverty-striken than any other age group. In 1971, this age group represented about 33 percent of the total population in the poverty continuum. Eight-million children under the age of 14 lived with families whose income was below the national poverty line. It must be remembered that those in this age group (as well as the parents or guardians) are unrepresented politically, economically, and socially. The primary reason for their economically impoverished status is simply the poverty of their parents.[10]

Although sex by itself does not represent a category of deprivation it is a significant factor of poverty when the main support of the family is the mother. Families headed by females fall substantially lower in the poverty continuum than do families headed by a man. There is a clear trend: more women are entering the labor force either as the main provider of support or to supplement the family's income. Employment and income for women are greatly affected by education, age, sex, family structure, and residential factors including availability of transportation.

With respect to family size, the traditional nuclear family with a planned number of children can lend itself to an optimal relationship between economic advantages and well-being of family members. When there are too many children in a family with a set income, which may be insufficient, a state of poverty exists.

The "psychology" of being poor, and the psychology of the poor, can best be understood in reference to the words of Michael Harrington: "There is, in short, a language of the poor, a psychology of the poor, a world view of the poor. To be impoverished is . . . to grow up in a culture that is radically different from the one that dominates society."[11] This status of being poor has also been called the "culture of poverty."

The Culture of Poverty

The culture of poverty includes the philosophy of the poor (how they view life, the present, and the future) and their living conditions. Like all other cultures, poverty tends to be passed on; it can be cyclic, may be self-perpetuating, and is assumed to be reinforced in the next generation. Being poor, some suggest, results in a certain life-style, which in turn contributes to a continuation of the state of poverty.

According to Oscar Lewis, many of the poor have beliefs, values, and life-styles that are not simply an adjustment to low income, but an ingrained way of life that is self-perpetuating and reinforced by each new generation. This life-style and status preclude both participation in community organizations and identification with the major institutions of society. Lewis generalizes that "people with a culture of poverty are provincial and locally oriented, they know only their troubles, their local conditions, their own neighborhood . . . they are not class conscious."[12]

According to this theory the poor are mired in despair and resignation, with a life-style that is characterized by fatalism, violence, unstable family structure, abandonment, and a total sense of the present. Lewis argues that poverty in itself may be brought under control. However, he goes on to state that the physical culture may not be so easily wiped out because "the elimination of poverty *per se* may not be enough to eliminate the culture of poverty."[13] That is, the cultural patterns of the poor are more important in their lives than is the condition of being poor. Lewis further contends that policy formulators intent on eliminating poverty must also abolish these life-styles and ways of perceiving the world and one's place in it if poverty is ever to be eradicated.

Critics of Lewis, Valentine[12] among them, point out that Lewis' concept of culture is contrary to the commonly accepted notion of culture in anthropology. Lewis conceives culture to be a total way of life of a particular group. Valentine and others object to the stance taken by proponents of the culture-of-poverty concept; they maintain that such investigators are biased by their own middle-class values and views of the poor. Valentine suggests that Lewis and those who think as he does fail to recognize other vital ethnic attributes of the Chicanos, Blacks, and other minorities that support their own way of life.

Much of what was planned and implemented during the 1960s—the decade billed as one of "rediscovery of poverty"—strove to break this poverty cycle through a variety of self-help and community-action programs. Essentially this was a comprehensive attack on most causes and aspects of poverty, with elimination of poverty as its unrealistic goal.

Cycle of Poverty and Poor Health:
The Medically Poor

The poor and the nearly poor have been excluded from the fee-for-medical-service system because of their inability to pay. Research has shown that the poor view their personal health as having low priority. "Health care ranks low on the poor man's list of priorities: if he feels passable today, he is less worried about the possibilities of seeing a doctor next week than he is about paying the rent tomorrow."[14] Statistically, in urban areas and where subsidized medical services for the poor have existed, the poor register a lower utilization rate than do people of the middle class. Yet the poor have higher disease rates than other groups. Underutilization of medical services by the poor and minorities has not been significantly altered in spite of the elimination of financial obstacles to relieve the economic burdens of the poor. In order to understand the causes of and factors related to this phenomenon of underutilization, the institutional and personal-access barriers to health care should be examined.[15]

Access barriers are identified as the following: language-communication isolation, poverty cycle, rural background of client when facing an urban medical institution, participation in seasonal migration patterns, sexism, institutional prejudice, and depersonalization.

The American health enterprise is basically a middle-class system, in which the major source of primary care is the private physician in group or solo practice with a fee-for-service method of payment. Physicians, for the most part, are from middle- or upper-class backgrounds and are unable or unwilling to practice in rural or urban ghetto areas where the poor reside. Consequently, they may lack knowledge about cultural and ethnic variances in needs actuated by illness and disease.

During the past ten years major expansion of medical-care facilities, manpower, and economic-assistance programs have become part of the medical enterprise. Medicare, Neighborhood Health Centers, various health-maintenance organizations, and allied health manpower have all had a part in altering the existing patterns of institutional exclusion of the poor. Although major gains were recorded in the availability and distribution of health services during this period, it appears that a familiar cycle of restrictiveness in delivery of health care is upon us. Consider, for example, the action taken in 1977 on both Federal and state levels to eliminate public funding for elective abortions for the poor and needy. Furthermore, health services for the poor have not expanded uniformly. Emphasis has been placed on specialized services, particularly birth control and out-patient mental-health services. For the poor and ghetto residents, acute episodic illnesses still mean a full day at a clinic—with the concomitant loss of income and/or time. General medical services attempted to expand and deliver health care in the form of comprehensive Neighborhood Health Centers. These facilities are government financed and are generally planned only for use by the poor. Unlike hospital out-patient departments and clinic settings, Neighborhood Health Centers were planned and developed to provide health care for the poor with a personal, ongoing relationship with physicians and other health personnel. Many health centers were created as a result of the racial riots of the middle 1960s. Since that time, Neighborhood Health Centers have become institutions that reflect community pride as well as centers of employment with considerable economic importance. Community residents have helped to overcome personal and institutional barriers to health-care services because of the personal nature of the medical care at these centers. In Neighborhood Health Centers in the Boston area, policy is generally the responsibility of the local citizens and their representative boards. Among the significant problem areas facing these health centers today are those of economics and manpower. Funding for these medical institutions has been drastically curtailed by the federal, state, and local governments, while costs on a per-patient basis have increased.

Earlier in this chapter, the characteristics of the poor were described in the context of the culture of poverty; these traits also include poor health. The cycle of poverty and poor health as shown in Figure 3 helps to explain the interlocking relationship between health and poverty. The most important components of this model are the relationships among resource allocation, environmental factors, medical-demand forces, biologic reproduction, public-health and morbidity factors, and social and psychological forces.

The relationship of resources, poverty, and health is a direct one. In our society, food, adequate shelter, clothing, and health care

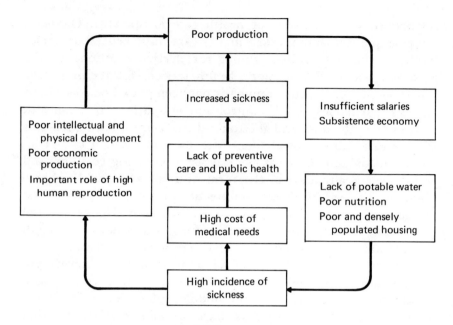

FIGURE 3.   The cycle of poverty and poor health.

are considered to be basic human needs, and are totally dependent on an individual's productivity. Resources include the economic
potential of the person and his family and the quality and quantity
of goods and services available to and affordable by the family.
Ideally, medical resources should be within easy access and affordable by all; they should also be of a comprehensive nature to
allow for total delivery of primary care. When insufficient wages
are earned, the need for medical services—unless it be for emergencies—must be weighted against other priorities such as food,
rent, utilities, and clothing.

Poor nutrition is considered to be a major health hazard in the
United States. For the poor, malnutrition and inadequate diet are
a very serious problem, especially among Blacks and Native Americans, closely followed by Spanish-speaking people and poor
whites.[16] The politics of nutrition in America continue to be
treated primarily as a problem of the poor, and the blame has been
directly but erroneously placed on their ignorance of proper
nutrition. Studies have shown that malnutrition is a leading cause
of infants' failure to thrive. Hunger is also a growing problem for
children and the elderly. Fixed incomes and the escalation of food

costs reduce the elderly to eat whatever may be within their purchasing power; it is no longer uncommon for the elderly to consume pet food. The provision of a daily "hot meal" in social-service centers and schools alleviates this nutritional problem somewhat; however, only a minority of the eligible elderly population and young people are reached through such programs. "Meals on wheels" is another example of nutritional assistance for the elderly shut-in. As our population grows increasingly older, nutritional deficits and chronic illness are becoming the most serious problems for the elderly. In the distinguished book by Nick Kotz, *Let Them Eat Promises,*[17] many cases are used to document the extent of the problem of hunger and malnutrition in America.

The relationship between housing and both physical and emotional health is supported by many studies of morbidity and disease in high-density living conditions. High density in housing units, rooms, and dwellings fosters impersonalization; social crowding correlates with high incidence of crime; high density can lead to schizophrenia and negative personal feelings of worth and alienation; and in most urban areas high density contributes to a higher incidence of illness and disease. Large cities with significant ghetto areas have reported several outbreaks of communicable diseases—diphtheria among them.[18] Large families are the norm with the poor and ethnic people of color, resulting in higher-than-normal density and overcrowded conditions that can result in the perpetuation of the cycle involving the pattern of culture, poverty, and poor health.

Another area that must be reckoned with in the model shown in Figure 3 is biologic reproduction. Reproductive forces and their relationship to the cycle of poverty and poor health are a subject of considerable discussion among those responsible for forming welfare policy. Reproductive forces include family planning with its concomitant availability, its effective use, the educational and economic status of the poor, and the achievement of desired family size. Numerous studies have shown a correlation among effective family planning, the actualization of ideal family size, socioeconomic status, and educational achievement. Race is also a factor: Black women whose socioeconomic status is low give birth to more children than they actually desire.[19] Obviously, the more children one has, the costlier it is to provide for their needs—such as education, food, health care, adequate housing, and cultural opportunities, to name only a few crucial necessities that middle- and upper-class people take for granted.

According to most experts, the most critical factor in biologic reproduction and achieving the ideal family size is education. The higher the educational achievement of both parents, the greater the chances are of reaching the desired family size (and the smaller the size of the family). Poor families by and large have a higher ratio of dependents—children and the elderly—and have the highest population growth trends in the United States. According to current demographic studies, future population growth in the United States is expected to come mostly from the Asian, Black, and Spanish ethnic and racial groups. This will occur among these particular groups because the concept of zero population growth has been understood, realized, and actively supported by the prevailing middle- and upper-socioeconomic classes in this country.

As shown in Figure 3, the allocation of medical services and manpower as well as the distribution of health care are directly linked to economic factors. Socioeconomic factors as well as demographic characteristics of a given population determine the availability, distribution, and consumption of medical services. The delivery system of health care also affects the demand because different subsystems deliver various levels of care (e.g., a physician's office versus a health clinic or a hospital). At the same time, demand and distribution forces are controlled by the medical profession. Most urban ghetto areas and sparsely settled rural areas are lacking in medical personnel and resources. The ever-growing medical and dental exodus to the well-to-do suburbs is a well-known fact. Private medical and dental practice in the core city is now a thing of the past. Most health services are currently being delivered in Neighborhood Health Centers or in hospital emergency rooms and/or clinics, where the cost factors are higher for the client than in private practice.

Medical demand affects the poor and minorities in another, more subtle manner. Ethnics and the poor are made "human diagnostic experimental objects" for the sake of medical advancement and medical education. The poor are also caught in the middle of the current dilemma regarding high cost of medical care versus benefit. Essentially the question is: Should expensive and experimental medical procedures be undertaken with any patient regardless of ability to pay or only with those who are able to pay? Whose life is worthy? Who decides? Resolution of such issues must be considered from a bioethical perspective. Needless to say, the unrepresented poor will continue to service medical practice and the medical establishment in a most supportive capacity.

There are other causes and consequences of poverty and poor health in the United States that include, as seen in Figure 3, public health, sanitation, and morbidity. Among the leading causes and factors of morbidity and death in the 1970s are cancer, heart disease, and accidents, which together account for more than two-thirds of all deaths. Clearly, life-style bears on the entire question. Statistically it has been supported that personal habits such as smoking and heavy drinking, as well as social conditions that cause tension, discord, poverty, and unemployment are all part and parcel of the disharmony between the individual and society. Elimination of physiologic and environmental causes of morbidity and mortality does not yet have social and political priority. In his 1950s study, Koos ascertained that the poor are not likely to make use of preventive health care because of personal problems and the impingement of more pressing priorities.[20]

Although there are those who argue that prevention is a myth, research has contributed immeasurably to the development of medication and tools used in primary prevention.[21] In the minds of many observers, it would seem that vaccinations, immunizations, and the use of antibiotics would make every disease curable. However, this viewpoint omits consideration of the relationship of disease to life-style. Personal health is seen by the poor mostly within a context of self-functioning and self-image.[22] Disability as a result of illness and disease is viewed as important only with respect to its effect on *social* functioning. Because of marginal employability, motivation to recover or recuperate in order to return to work is not high. Psychological barriers in this cycle of poverty and poor health further involve the inability to delay gratification (a value cherished by middle-class, work-oriented people), a socially determined difference in personality structure, alienation from society at large, and institutional racism. The relationship between the forces that directly affect both the socio-psychological and morbidity status of the poor must be carefully examined and reevaluated by health-care providers.

PROGRAMS TO HELP THE POOR

Echoing Harrington's earlier-cited study of 1963, most official governmental agencies and human-service institutions responsible for planning and providing social, economic, and health services for the poor note that approximately 1 out of 5 Americans is living with incomes below the poverty line. This line is generally drawn at $5,500 for a nonrural family of four, with about $12,000 being necessary to maintain a no-frill standard of living in cities such as Boston, New York, San Francisco, Houston, Honolulu, and Atlanta.* For most minorities, the elderly, and the poor, this figure is far out of reach. Who are these impersonally treated poor, and how are they expected to survive? How are they expected to achieve a decent standard of living and health?

In the 1960s the "War on Poverty" was promoted as a solution to the socioeconomic distress found in this nation. The Economic Opportunity Act of 1964 was regarded as the beginning of an all-out campaign to eradicate poverty. Like many other federal programs, the new law was created to attack the basic causes of poverty. It sought to provide ways for the poor to lift themselves out of the depths of despair and take advantage of the opportunities already available to them, thus emphasizing the notion of self-help. The act underestimated the deep-seated racist attitudes that excluded minorities from receiving a sufficient education, adequate housing, full employment, and ready access to health care, services for children, and improved nutrition. And in the health field, few in policy-making positions or in health services acknowledged that "there has been developed a broad recognition that health is a vital concern. It is generally recognized by the Western countries that medical care should be made available to all people, regardless of their ability to pay, thereby bringing the best quality of care to them when they need it."[23]

A major goal of antipoverty legislation was to coordinate, at all levels of government, Federal agencies with services and resources related to poverty and to enable the poor to become the beneficiaries. It was recognized that the poor were not taking advantage of the various Federal and state programs available to

*Department of Labor statistics, 1976.

them. The program was aimed primarily at the very young, through educational and training opportunities, in the hope of eliminating poverty in the next generation. The central focus was to strive for the fullest possible involvement of the poor in planning, developing, and implementing such programs. By giving the poor opportunities to learn and develop marketable skills, the Office of Economic Opportunity (OEO) expected that people would be able to secure jobs and improve their employment condition and that the entrenched cycle of poverty would thus come to an end. At that time a series of forward-looking programs were generated by OEO. In the field of education and special training, the most important programs were the Neighborhood Youth Corps, Job Corps, Adult Basic Education, and Work Experience and Training. In the area of economics and finance there were loans made available to small businesses and rural areas. The most visible and well-supported program was the Community Action Program (CAP), which promoted neighborhood service centers, Neighborhood Health Centers, Head Start, legal services for the poor, and family planning programs. Volunteers in Service to America (VISTA) and small-scale programs to aid migrant laborers and their families were also created by the Economic Opportunity Act. The Model Cities program also owes its inception to the concept of participatory democracy: giving the poor a greater voice in controlling program decisions, resources, and activities.[24]

In 1969, when Richard Nixon became president, major changes in the Johnson-era, human-service programs for the poor were anticipated. By his second term in office, President Nixon had either eliminated, transferred to other departments, or minimized the funding of successful programs. According to the promoters of Nixon's "creative federalism," individual success and self-improvement were to be achieved through self-help, not through governmental intervention or handouts.

Community-Action Program

This program was designed to attack the forces that perpetuate and/or cause poverty. It proposed that all local resources would work together in a coordinated way to improve local conditions that keep people poor. In order to accomplish this, community-action agencies (CAAs) were organized in each community and were to be independent from all local governmental agencies. Participation in the CAP agency was to be open to all local residents, and they in turn were required to exert "maximum feasible participation" in all programs and ultimately in making all decisions. Citizen participation was taken to mean local decision making by representative boards elected from the community. In many cases, local community decisions were in conflict with those of the established political bodies, and this led to open conflict between the community residents and public agencies and officials. For the poor, this program meant control of their own destinies and an end to their political, social, and economic powerlessness. By 1971 there were over 900 CAAs around the country. Each agency was charged with the mission of providing services appropriate to local poverty needs. Another responsibility of the CAA was that of refining the "goals of Community Action by influencing other institutions and by enhancing its own capacity to respond creatively to new poverty situations and traditional methods of dealing with them."[25] To carry out the service component of the antipoverty mission, CAAs established more than 3000 neighborhood service centers in poor communities. Many Neighborhood Health Centers were also established to provide for the health needs of the poor and minorities in medically underserved urban and ghetto areas.

Evaluation of the CAP and CAAs indicates that a small number of the hardcore poor has been reached. Some claim that the program has done little more than to take the cream off the top of the low-income population, helping those who are perhaps least in need of help. Others have charged that the local programs have not affected the real basis of poverty and maintain that the services they give are only rehabilitative in nature.[26]

Among the most lasting and important contributions of this program has been a fostering of local pride and the training of local residents who have subsequently secured employment as paraprofessionals—such as teacher's aids, nurses' aids, community outreach workers, and mental-health and laboratory aids. Through these jobs and training programs many local poor have been able to advance toward a professional career.

Head Start

This program was one of the most popular initiated by OEO. Head Start was developed to provide the early development of vocabulary skills, cultural experiences, and intellectual stimulation denied disadvantaged children and enjoyed by children from more affluent families. Medical and psychological examinations as well as other specialized health and dental-care programs and social services were provided in many cases for the first time.

Legal Services and Other Programs

Although legal services for the poor are available through Legal Aid Societies, too few of these agencies exist and poor people avoid using them. Legal services are located in the neighborhoods of the poor and are staffed by attorneys who work full time and provide free legal services to the poor. The majority of legal problems brought to such agencies are in the areas of domestic and family relations, protection from regulatory agencies, and use of general consumer laws.

Other programs planned and implemented by OEO were vocational training and educational opportunities for the youth. Another direct effort of OEO was the Special Emphasis programs—directed mainly toward Native Americans (Indians), the elderly, migrants, and rural families. In 1971, OEO estimated that of every 100 people 65 or older, 30 are poor; of every 100 Indians living on reservations, 80 are poor. For city dwellers the figure is in the high 80s; for migrant laborers, it is 90. For the United States as a whole, OEO estimated that 13 of every 100 are poor (according to standard measures of poverty).[27]

SUMMARY AND CONCLUSIONS

Poverty in America is by no means a new phenomenon, although the realization that it constitutes a *major* social problem that demands public attention and governmental action is new. There are two reasons for the new status of poverty as a public issue and social concern.

The most important factor is the growing realization that poverty is not an individual problem but a societal one. We no longer assume that anyone can become an economic success in America or that those who fail to do so have only themselves to blame. Some persons who are living in poverty in these decades cannot and should not be in the labor force because of physical disability or family conditions (e.g., welfare mothers or the very elderly).

Second, as our society becomes more affluent, poverty becomes more noticeable and harmful. We now see the deeply felt effects of poverty in maintaining each generation of individuals and families in a cycle. Hunger and poor nutrition exist in a land that pays producers to grow less or to create surpluses at the expense of many who are victims of our stratified society.

One result of poverty's greater "visibility" has been a myriad of social programs that started in the 1960s, and which are discussed in this chapter. It should be pointed out that poverty and the concomitant dependency of those who are impoverished have *not* been reduced thus far.

It seems that poverty has always been with us and, unfortunately, will remain with us for years to come. But it is also evident that poverty—as well as affluence and good health—is a human-made condition that human efforts and planning can change for the better. Any intervention affects each person and the poverty-producing factors differently. Psychological factors, however, present a different set of problems: ones tied to the socialization process and hence part of the generation cycle. These effects are not so amenable to rapid change and intervention. The hard-to-reach, multiproblem family has been observed in social work and medical practice and has been described in the literature for quite a long time because of its conspicuous reluctance to change its way of life under professional guidance.[28] As suggested elsewhere throughout this book, it behooves the health-care provider to reach a clearer understanding of, and appreciation for, the multifaceted aspects of cultural and ethnic diversity that may act in concert with the effects of poverty.

Individual independence from others for common human needs—whether medical, economic, political, cultural or psychological—will be our next battle.

REFERENCES

1. John Kosa, "Chapter 1 in" *Poverty and Health: A Sociological Analysis,* ed. John Kosa, Aaron Antonovsky, and Irving K. Zola (Cambridge: Harvard University Press, 1969), pp. 1-33.
2. *The New York Times,* 17 July, 1977.
3. John K. Galbraith, *The Affluent Society* (Boston: Houghton Mifflin, 1958), pp. 322-325.
4. Michael Harrington, *The Other America: Poverty in the United States* (New York: Macmillan, 1972).
5. *The New York Times,* 17 July, 1977.
6. Ibid.
7. Ibid.
8. Ibid.
9. Mark G. Arnold and Greg Rosenbaum, *The Crime of Poverty* (Skokie, Ill.: National Text Book, 1973), p. 16.
10. Ibid., p. 17.
11. Harrington, op. cit.[4]
12. Charles Valentine, *Culture and Poverty* (Chicago: University of Chicago Press, 1968)
13. Ibid., p. 73.
14. *Health in America: 1776-1976* (Washington, D.C.: U.S. Department of Health, Education, and Welfare Health Resources Administration, 1976), p. 176.
15. Manuel Spector and Rachel Spector, "Access Barriers to Health Care for the Spanish-Speaking in the Urban Setting" (presented at the American Public Health Association Annual Meeting, Miami, October 16-21, 1976).
16. *Minority Health Chart Book* (Washington, D.C.: American Public Health Association, 1974) p. 49.
17. Nick Kotz, *Let Them Eat Promises* (New York: Doubleday, 1971).
18. Bonnie Bullough and Vern Bullough, *Poverty, Ethnic Identity and Health Care* (New York: Appleton, 1972), p. 58.
19. Arthur A. Campbell, "Fertility and Family Planning among Non-White Married Couples in the United States," *Eugenics Quarterly* 12 (September 1961): 124-131.
20. Earl L. Koos, *Health in Regionville* (New York: Columbia University Press, 1954).
21. Manuel Spector and Rachel Spector, "Prevention: Myth or Reality?" *Health Education* 8 (July/August 1977): 23-25.
22. E. Suchmann, "Socio-Medical Variations among Ethnic Groups," *American Journal of Sociology* 70 (November 1964): 319-331.
23. *Health in America: 1776-1976,*[14] p. 172.
24. Office of Economic Opportunity Pamphlet, Office of Operations, 000-2 (Washington, D.C.: U.S. Government Printing Office, 1971), p. 2.

25. "Special Programs," Office of Economic Opportunity Pamphlet 6.100-1 (Washington, D.C.: U.S. Government Printing Office, 1971).
26. Ferne Dolodner, "Community Action: Where Has It Been? Where Will It Go?" *Annals of the American Academy of Political Science* 385 (September 1969): 36-40.
27. "Special Programs."[25]
28. H. S. Takvlia et al., *The Health Center Doctor in India* (Baltimore: Johns Hopkins University Press, 1967).

BIBLIOGRAPHY: POVERTY: THE BARRIER TO HEALTH CARE

Arnold, Mark G., and Rosenbaum, Greg. *The Crime of Poverty.* Skokie, Ill.: National Textbook, 1973.

This book presents an overview of reasons for the failure of the war on poverty. It is written in the context of what it means to be poor in contemporary American society. It also explores methods that poor people can employ to help themselves out of poverty.

De Castro, Josue. *The Black Book of Hunger.* Boston: Beacon Press, 1967.

Topics such as the relationship between hunger and the economic imbalance of the world, the fight against hunger, and the world association for the struggle against hunger are discussed. Good reference.

Feagin, Joe R. *Subordinating the Poor: Welfare and American Beliefs.* Englewood Cliffs, N.J.: Prentice-Hall, 1975.

Feagin explodes the common American myths about poverty and the welfare system and describes how these erroneous beliefs evolved. The book also demonstrates how these beliefs have become tools to keep the poor in their place and preserve the economic and social status quo.

Freire, Paulo. *Pedagogy of the Oppressed.* Translated by Myra Bugman Ramos. New York: The Seabury Press, 1970.

This study of education explores topics such as the contradiction between the oppressors and the oppressed and how it is overcome. It describes the use of education as an instrument for liberation.

Gordon, David M. *Theories of Poverty and Underemployment.* Lexington, Mass.: Heath, 1972.

The reader will discover a complex analysis of the various economic factors and theories that explain poverty. The theories of poverty and underemployment—orthodox economic theory, dual labor and market theory, and radical economic theory—are freely discussed and compared.

Hickel, Walter J. *Who Owns America?* New York: Paperback Library, 1972.

Hickel describes the deception and lack of self-confidence within the Nixon Administration; how environmental decisions that affect life in America are made, and by whom.

Kain, John F., editor. *Race and Poverty: The Economics of Discrimination.* Englewood Cliffs, N.J.: Prentice-Hall, 1969.

The two major issues confronting American society are discussed. This book explores both areas and their interrelationships.

Kosa, John, and Zola, Irving Kenneth. *Poverty and Health: A Sociological Analysis*, 2nd ed. Cambridge, Mass.: Harvard University Press, 1976.

This book explores areas such as the nature of poverty, social aspects of health and illness, prevention of illness and maintenance of health, and the future of poverty.

Kotz, Nick. *Let Them Eat Promises.* Garden City, N.Y.: Doubleday, 1971.

Kotz provides an excellent description of the politics of hunger in the United States. The book begins with the "discovery of hunger" and explores the actions and inactions that surround this issue.

Mandell, Betty Reid, editor. *Welfare in America: Controlling the "Dangerous Classes."* Englewood Cliffs, N.J.: Prentice-Hall, 1975.

Explored are issues such as how social-welfare services are "often designed not to help the poor but to keep them in their places."

Piven, Frances Fox, and Cloward, Richard A. *Regulating the Poor: The Functions of Public Welfare.* New York: Vintage Books, 1971.

This book is about relief-giving and how it is used to regulate the political and economic behavior of the poor. It seeks to explain why welfare exists and why the welfare rolls expand and contract.

Roby, Pamela, editor. *The Poverty Establishment.* Englewood Cliffs, N.J.: Prentice-Hall, 1974.

From this anthology one gains some insight into the power structure that not only creates but maintains poverty programs to regulate the poor and preserve inequality by continuously generating ways to increase the power and profits of the wealthy.

Shostak, Arthur B.; Van Til, Jon; and Van Til, Sally Bould. *Privilege in Ameri-*

ca: An End to Inequality? Englewood Cliffs, N.J.: Prentice-Hall, 1973.

This book describes various aspects of an ancient human dream—the reduction of social inequality. The first section of the book explores the major ways in which equality and inequality are explained and justified, and the third section examines specific programs aimed at the reduction of inequality.

Trattner, Walter I. *From Poor Law to Welfare State: A History of Social Welfare in America.* New York: Free Press, 1974.

Trattner has compiled an outstanding, comprehensive history of social welfare in the United States. The book presents the developments of welfare from colonial times to the present and the milieu in which each policy change took place.

Valentine, Charles A. *Culture and Poverty.* Chicago: University of Chicago Press, 1968.

This work goes beyond what has been written about the poor and their ways of life. It contains commentary on social problems and questions of value judgements related to poverty.

FURTHER SUGGESTED READINGS

Books

Fry, John. *Locked Out Americans.* New York: Harper, 1973.

Galbraith, John K. *The Affluent Society.* Boston: Houghton Mifflin, 1958.

Gottlieb, D., and Heinsohn, Anne. *America's Other Youth Growing Up Poor.* Englewood Cliffs, N.J.: Prentice-Hall, 1970.

Harrington, Michael. *The Other American: Poverty in the United States.* New York: Macmillan, 1962.

Minuchin, S.; Montalvo, B; Guerney, Jr., B; Rosman, B; and Schumer, F. *Families of the Slums.* New York: Basic Books, 1967.

Articles

Campbell, Archie A. "Fertility and Family Planning among Non-White Married Couples in the United States." *Eugenics Quarterly* 12 (September 1961): 124-131.

Dolodner, Ferne. "Community Action: Where Has It Been? Where Will it Go?" *Annals of the American Academy of Political Science* 385 (September 1969): 36-40.

Humphrey, Patricia. "Learning about Poverty and Health." *Nursing Outlook* 22 (July 1974): 441-443.

Suchman, Edward, "Socio-Medical Variables among Ethnic Groups." *American Journal of Sociology* 70 (November 1964): 319-331.

"The Sick Poor": Supplemental Section to the *American Journal of Nursing* 69 (November 1969): 2423-2454. Includes: English, J. T., "The Dimensions of Poverty;" Geiger, H. J., "The Endlessly Revolving Door;" Mahoney, M. E., "Momentum for Change;" McNeary, W. S., "Changing the Health Care System."

CHAPTER 8
Is Health Care
a Right?

Before you begin to read this chapter, please answer the following questions:

1. What is meant by a right?
2. Whose right takes precedence over whose right—the consumer's or the provider's?
3. Is the concern primarily with the right of access to health care or with the right to free care?
4. How will free health care affect the health-care delivery system in general? How will it affect *your* practice specifically?
5. a. Will health care improve if it is free?
   b. Will it improve health status? Longevity? Quality of life? If yes, how? If no, how?
6. Will health care mandated by federal law be provided with dignity, or will a bad situation (i.e., inequalities in health care) get worse?
7. Is part of the difficulty with health-care delivery an inability of the consumer to (a) wade through the layers of the health-care system and/or (b) understand the jargon of the health-care system?
8. What, if any, methods could be applied to alter the problems of health-care delivery?
9. Even if health is recognized as a right, do not *people* have the ultimate responsibility or power to protect this right?
10. What is meant by government control?
11. Is health the property or responsibility of the state?

Let us assume that a belief underlying our professional practice is that health care is a right. What does such a philosophy mean? This fundamental issue has been widely debated over the past several years. Since the concept led to the creation of a national health policy, it continues to be the focal point of numerous questions. Furthermore, it forms a key issue in this book: the philosophical link between the worlds of the provider and of the consumer.

The following two subchapters provide a background for the affirmative and negative positions. Presented here is an editorially revised version of the text of a debate between Hildegarde Peplau, a distinguished nursing leader, representing the affirmative, and Robert Sade, a physician who has attained national attention through his articles and oratory delineating the arguments against health care as a right. This debate was sponsored by Sigma Theta Tau (National Nursing Honor Society) at Boston College in October, 1972. It remains a classic representation of the opposing views of this critical issue.

Negative Response

Robert Sade

Over the past 40 years the proportion of the nation's wealth expended for health care has more than doubled, from 3.6 percent of the Gross National Product in 1929 to 7.4 percent in 1971. Much more significant than that rise, however, is the fact that, during the same period, the proportion of health expenditures coming from public sources rose 400 percent—from 8.9 percent in 1929 to 35.8 percent in 1971. In the last fiscal year, the federal government spent more than $26 billion on health care. Depending on which of many current plans before the Congress is adopted, that figure could rise toward $100 billion over the next few years. The massiveness of government health expenditures is illustrated by the fact that in 1970 the Department of Health, Education, and Welfare alone spent $9 billion more than the total of all the profits made by all the corporations in the United States.

Something very big is happening to American medicine. It is being engulfed by a giant leviathan that at times seems irresistible. The fuel that powers the federal leviathan is public support for its health goal: the nationalization of medicine. Yet that popular support is irrational and did not arise spontaneously. It was pro-

Revised from an article in *Image* 7 (February 1974): 11-19. Specific references for quoted material were not provided.

duced by demogoguery. A University of Chicago study last year showed that 75 percent of heads of families believe that there is a "crisis" in medical care at this time, and 75 percent believe that Federal control of the health industry, based on a Medicare pattern, would bring better medical care for people of low or moderate income. In the same sampling, only 10 percent of those questioned were unhappy with the overall quality of their own health care. This marked discrepancy between personal experience with health care and beliefs regarding the health care of others can have arisen from only one source: misrepresentations by persons with very powerful public voices.

If misplaced public support is the fuel that powers the federal health leviathan, then the heart that gives the creature life and makes its existence possible is the Big Lie. This Big Lie is the one that has made all the others possible, the one that has reversed the roles of thief and victim, the one that penalizes productiveness, rewards mediocrity, and sneers at justice: the concept that health care is a right. I will briefly consider the meaning of the word *right* and then present some of the ways in which the perversion of that concept has been implemented politically around the world.

A *right* defines a freedom of action. For instance, a right to a material object is the uncoerced choice of the use to which that object will be put; a right to a specific action, such as free speech, is the freedom to engage in the activity without forceful repression. The moral foundation of the rights of man begins with the fact that he is a living creature; he has the right to his own life. All other rights are corollaries of this primary one; without the right to life, there can be no others.

> . . . for every individual, a right is the moral sanction of a positive—of his freedom to act on his own judgment, for his own goals, by his own voluntary uncoerced choice. As to his neighbors, his rights impose no obligations on them except of a negative kind: to abstain from violating his rights.

The freedom to live does not automatically ensure life. For man, a specific course of action is required in order to sustain his life, a course of action that must be guided by reason and reality and that has as its goal the creation or acquisition of material objects, such as food and clothing, and intellectual values, such as self-esteem and integrity. His moral system is the means by which he is able to select those values that will support his life and allow him to achieve his happiness.

The right to life implies three corollaries: first, the right to select those values one deems necessary to sustain one's own life; second, the right to exercise one's own judgment of the best course of action to achieve the chosen values; and third, the right to dispose of those values, once gained, in any way one chooses, without coercion by other men. The denial of any one of these corollaries severely compromises or destroys the right to life itself. A man who is not allowed to choose his own goals, is prevented from setting his own course in achieving those goals, and is not free to dispose of the values he has earned is no less than a slave to those who usurp those rights. The right to private property, therefore, is essential and indispensable to maintaining free men in a free society.

In a free society, man exercises his right to sustain his own life by producing economic values in the form of goods and services that he is, or should be, free to exchange with other men who are similarly free to trade or not trade with him. The economic values produced, however, are not given as gifts by nature, but exist only by virture of the thought and effort of individual men. Goods and services are thus owned as a consequence of the right to sustain life by one's own physical and mental effort.

It is the nature of man as a living, thinking being that determines his natural rights. The concept of human rights, or natural rights, was introduced to the civilized world by Aristotle, who spoke of natural justice and of equal treatment before the law for all men, while noting that unequal merit should result in unequal reward. Thomas Aquinas expanded Aristotle's work by describing the existence of a natural law from which arose natural rights. These rights were recognized as prior to and existing apart from positive law: "Written law indeed contains natural right, but it does not institute it, for its force comes, not from the law, but from nature."

One of the most important defenders of human rights was John Locke, who was quite explicit as to what these rights were:

> The law of nature . . . which obliges everyone, and reason which is that law, teaches all mankind who will but consult

> it, that being all equal and independent, no one ought to
> harm another in his life, health, liberty, or possessions.

In direct line of intellectual succession to Locke were Thomas
Jefferson and the founders of the American republic. The Declaration of Independence speaks of "inalienable rights," and the
Constitution of 1787 made the United States the first major
government founded on the explicit proposition that the rights
of the people are not granted by the state, but arise from the
nature of man, and are beyond the right of the state either to
grant or to withhold:

> We hold these truths to be self-evident: that all men are
> created equal; that they are endowed by their Creator with
> certain inalienable rights; that among these are life, liberty,
> and the pursuit of happiness.

One of the models for the Declaration of Independence was the
Bill of Rights for Virginia, which contained this statement:

> All men are born equally free and independent and have
> certain inherent rights—among which are enjoyment of life,
> liberty, and pursuing and obtaining happiness and safety.

The only fundamental change in this idea when it was incorporated
in the Declaration of Independence was in Jefferson's realization
that there is no right to obtain happiness; there is only the right
to pursue it.

Since 1787, conceptual clarity in the consideration of rights has
been gradually lost. As great a jurist as Justice Oliver Wendell
Homes remarked that "a right is but a prophecy that the state
will use its course and its might to sustain a man's claim." The
greatest perversion of the concept of rights occurred during the
presidency of Franklin Delano Roosevelt, when *right* was
surreptitiously transferred from the freedom to pursue a value
to the value itself: now all Americans had the right to a job, the
right to a house, the right to a clean this and a decent that. The
day of "natural rights" was gone, and the "parasite rights" of the
New Deal crept up in the night.

As if dissatisfied with the rape and mutilation of the idea of
rights, modern politicians have now reduced it to utter absurdity.

The Democrats, in their 1972 platform, promised to secure the right of the American people to health—not to health care, but to health itself: "Good Health is the least this society should promise its citizens. We endorse the principle that good health is a right of all Americans." If they thought it would make political hay, no doubt they would also promise to secure the inherent right of the people to good looks and superior intelligence.

In fact, there is a limited, specific sense in which health may be thought of as a right. It is that no man may harm the health of another, under sanction of the same moral force protecting the right to life. To invert the logic of rights and claim that there is an obligation upon society to provide health for its citizens not only is logically absurd and morally indefensible, but is also medically impossible. Statistics from the Department of Health, Education, and Welfare show that last year 67 percent of deaths were due to diseases known to be caused or exacerbated by alcohol, tobacco smoking, and overeating or were due to accidents. Each of these factors is either largely or wholly correctable by individual action. Many common illnesses have a relationship like that of mortality to personal habits and excesses. We could, of course, make alcohol and tobacco illegal, prescribe diets for everyone (to be enforced by the FBI and FDA as a joint project), and put an end to airplanes and automobiles. The history of the Eighteenth Amendment in particular and of Western civilization in general should not stop us. After all, the Health of the Nation is at stake.

The concept of medical care as the patient's right is immoral because it denies the most fundamental of all rights: that of a man to his own life and the freedom of action to support it. Medical care is neither a right nor a privilege; it is a service that is provided by physicians and others to people who wish to purchase it. It is the provision of the service that a physician depends on for his livelihood and is his means of supporting his own life.

The very question of whether health care is a right or a privilege is an invalid one, because it is based on an erroneous supposition. The word *privilege* is derived from the Latin *privus*, private, and *lex*, law, forming the word *privilegium*, which means "a law for or against a private person." A privilege is a "right or immunity granted as a peculiar benefit or favor." The fallacy of the right-or-a-privilege question is revealed by rephrasing the question: Should health care be granted to a limited number of people (as a privilege), or should it be granted to everyone (as a right)? This question should properly be answered by two questions: Granted by whom? And at whose expense? The answers are: granted by an arbitrary coercive agency, the government, at the expense of every tax-payer and every health professional. Health care cannot morally be granted to anyone. It is a service that must be treated as any other service: it must be purchased by those who wish to buy it or given as a gift to the sick by the only human beings who are competent to give that gift—the health professionals themselves.

Starting with the notion that medical care is a right, it is argued that the right must be secured for the people, that anything that must be paid for is not a right, and that the government must therefore provide free medical care for its citizens. The electorate that has been taught that money is evil, that living far beyond one's income is suicidal for an individual, but perfectly acceptable for a government, that the product of a man's labor is fair game for expropriation by his fellow citizens—such people believe that medical care can be made free.

"There ain't no such thing as a free lunch." There is no such thing as free medical care. "'Health care is purchasable,' meaning that somebody has to pay for it, individually or collectively, at the expense of foregoing the current or future consumption of other things." The question is whether the decision of how to allocate the consumer's dollar should belong to the consumer or to the state. I have already shown that the choice of how a doctor's services should be rendered belongs only to the doctor; in the same way, the choice of whether to buy a health service rather than some other service or commodity belongs to the consumer as a logical consequence of the right to his own life.

Ignoring the irrationality and logical inconsistencies of its own programs, the government rushes forth to secure the right of its people to health care. In order to protect their basic human rights, that is, in order to protect themselves from violence perpetrated on them by other men, people form governments and invest their governments with a monopoly of the use of force. The government can use force for only one purpose—to retaliate against those who initiate violence. In serving as the repository for the retaliatory use of force, the government serves its only moral purpose—the protection of human rights. Governments, though, have not always stayed within those bounds, despite the most stringent constitutional safeguards. As a matter of fact, they have never stayed within those bounds. Fascination with the fact that power corrupts has provided the world with some of its greatest literature.

The degree to which a government exercises its monopoly on the retaliatory use of force by asserting a claim to the lives and property of its citizens is the degree to which it has eroded its own legitimacy. It is a frequently overlooked fact that behind every law is a policeman's gun or a soldier's bayonet. When that gun and bayonet are used to initiate violence, to take property, or to restrict liberty by force, there are no longer any rights, for the lives of the citizens belong to the state.

Any act of force is anti-mind. It is a confession of the failure of persuasion and the failure of reason. When politicians say that the health system must be forced into a mold of their own design, they are admitting their inability to persuade doctors and patients to use the plan voluntarily; they are proclaiming the supremacy of the state's logic over the judgments of the individual minds of all concerned with health care. Statists throughout history have never learned that compulsion and reason are contradictory, that a forced mind cannot think effectively and, by extension, that a regimented profession will eventually choke and stagnate from its own lack of freedom.

The immorality of all legislative acts that are based on the principle of health care as a right is best illustrated by noting their effects on a group that will be most affected by nationalization of the health care industry—physicians. Remembering that doctors are also citizens and as such have the same rights as all other citizens, we may note that any doctor who is forced by law to join a group or hospital he does not choose, or is prevented by law from prescribing a drug he thinks is best for his patient, or is compelled by law to make any decision he would not otherwise have made, is being forced to act against his own mind, which means forced to act against his own life. He is also being forced to violate his most fundamental professional commitment—that of using his own best judgment at all times for the maximal benefit of his patient.

These acts of force against physicians are attacks on very basic political principles. If they are allowed to pass unprotested, they can be, and probably will be, used against every other citizen or group of citizens in the country. The right to health care is clearly the instrument of a political movement seeking a common goal— the nationalization of the health care industry or, put in a more descriptive term, the socialization of medicine. If this goal were to be reached, do we have any indication of what would happen to health care in the United States? Lacking a crystal ball to reveal the future, we can best see forward by looking backward, to historical precedent. Both political and economic histories abound with warnings of what is to come.

Regulation of health care services by the state began with the passage of Bismarck's Sickness Insurance Law in 1883. The purpose of that law was to preempt the growing political power of the new German socialist movement by mollifying the working people with a paternalistic medical program. The purely political goals associated with the passage of medical legislation in most countries have usually been attained: consolidation of political power by giving "free" goods or services to the electorate. Political goals have rarely been explicit. Instead, the reasons given for nationalization have related to improvement of health of the people and can be divided into three general categories: the improvement of the quality of health care; providing care to more people by expansion of personnel and facilities; and the improvement of the overall health of the nation, as measured by standard health indices. None of these nonpolitical goals has been consistently achieved by any nation merely by legislatively controlling its health-care industry.

Measurement of the quality of medical care has always been an ephemeral undertaking. There are no generally accepted criteria for achieving this measurement. Many recent attempts to quantitate "quality" by the manipulation of various statistical data have been as uniformly unsuccessful as the contradiction implicit in quality versus quantity. There are, however, a number of indirect indicators of quality of medical care that have been studied with respect to the presence or absence of government control of medicine in a variety of countries.

The foundation of excellence in medical care is the doctor-patient relationship. Before the advent of scientific medicine in the nineteenth century, most of the good that doctors did for patients was accomplished as a direct result of the esteem in which the doctor was held, the trust that the patient had in his judgment, the respect that the physician had for his patient as a human being, and the manner in which that respect was projected. The fact that there are now some diseases that can be cured as a result of the application of the scientific method to human disease does not diminish the importance of the art of medicine in achieving salutary results in treatment. The art of medicine cannot be practiced without a large measure of mutual confidence, that is, the highest possible level of doctor-patient relationship.

This relationship is attacked and eroded from virtually every side with increasing government control of medicine. Although it is impossible to assign numerical values to a subjective phenomenon such as this, a survey of seven major nations uncovered several mechanisms by which bureaucratization undermines the doctor-patient relationship. The undermining factors include a decrease in time available to establish rapport due to the increase in both patient load and paper work for physicians. There is an erosion of mutual trust between physician and patient. The patient recognizes that the records being kept of his illness are not confidential but available for scrutiny by bureaucrats whose job it is to ensure efficient and frugal operation of the system. The physician, because he is paid by the state, is assigned a central role in protecting the solvency of the system by uncovering malingering and assigning benefits of the system as an agent of the state rather than as servant of the patient.

An eloquent description of the nature of the doctor-patient relationship in a country with a well-developed socialized medical system comes from a Russian physician:

> The largest part of the ten minutes allocated as the norm for a patient's visit is consumed in writing.
>
> And the patient? How do you think he feels when he walks into the physician's office with his ailments and sees that the doctor's attention is riveted not to the person but to the papers? Questions are asked abruptly. At times the patient's answers reach the doctor's ears but not his consciousness.
>
> Listening to the complaints with one ear and with his head bent over his papers, writing, the doctor sometimes does not even look at his patient . . . .
>
> Late at night the doctor returns home, barely dragging his weary limbs, and starts to write what he had not been able to put down during the day while he was with his patients. . . .

> As for the patient, he is not so much treated as "officially processed."
> Under the present system, consideration and concern for the sick patient sink into the background. The very process of medical thought is bureaucratized. The doctor-thinker is transformed into the doctor-bureaucrat.

To gain the trust of his patient, the physician must project a sense of interest in his patient's illness. The loss of interest in his work was described by a Swedish physician as he wrote of the effects (on Swedish physicians) of the nationalization of Swedish medicine:

> The details and the implicated working schedule have not yet been determined in all hospitals and districts, but the general feeling of belonging to a free profession, free to decide—at least in principle—how to organize its work, has been lost. Many hospital-based physicians regard their work now with an apathy previously unknown.

The reduction of time available to develop rapport and treat sick patients has occurred virtually everywhere that state medicine has been introduced. In Germany, the average office visit in panel practice is six minutes, and the number of patients seen in one day varies between 50 and 100. The average visit in Britain of 12 minutes includes traveling time for house calls, finding and filing patients' cards, entering clerical details and issuing certificates, history taking, time for the patient to dress and undress, clinical examination, and time for thought and advising the patient. In Sweden the situation is just as bad. In out-patient departments of hospitals, which do 40 percent of all open (outside-hospital) medical care:

> . . . the great number of patients to be treated in a short time gives rise to a type of activity that excludes personal contact. Patients complain of long waiting hours, of disrupted diagnostic procedures, of lack of privacy, and above all the difficulty of getting assurance of continuous treatment by the same doctor and a good heart-to-heart talk with him. They feel like numbered objects put into a complicated machine, where a doctor—any doctor—is one of the cogs among all the technical niceties and laboratory procedures.

The quality of medical care cannot improve when some providers of that care, physicians, are demonstrably dissatisfied and unhappy with their professional lot. Professional discontent has been manifested in many ways. Work strikes by physicians are unheard of in any country until government intervenes in the profession. Strikes against government-imposed conditions have occurred in many countries—for instance, in Austria in 1955, Sweden in 1957, again in Austria in 1962, Belgium in 1963, Saskatchewan in 1964, and Japan in 1970. The discontent of physicians in Britain since the institution of the National Health Service (NHS) in 1948 is well known. Since the inception of the NHS, dozens of committees and commissions have been formed because of belated recognition of some aspects of professional discontent. One extremely effective way for a physician to demonstrate his unhappiness is to leave his own country for one in which he will be better able to achieve his professional goals. This effect of socialization on the medical profession is best demonstrated by the emigration phenomenon that took place in Britain following the inception of the NHS. During the first 15 years of the NHS, 600 British physicians, or one-third of the output of the medical schools of the United Kingdom and Ireland, settled abroad every year, and the rate of emigration of physicians was five times what it was in the 1930s. This astounding desertion of the homeland was not simply part of the well-known "brain-drain" in England, since the medical emigration rate during that time period was six times the general emigration rate. The fact that the emigration rate has now slowed somewhat is probably a reflection of the selection of persons entering the profession who are more willing to work under the restrictive and stultifying atmosphere of medical practice that has been produced by the NHS.

High-quality medical care requires more than a good doctor-patient relationship and contented physicians. It also requires a sound scientific foundation and an active program of basic medical and biological research. Making available billions of dollars' worth of braces, orthopedic appliances, and reconstructive operations to thousands of victims of polio can be accomplished in the short run by political manipulation of the medical system. A far more significant achievement is the isolation of the polio virus and the immunization of an entire population against it, completely wiping out the disease. This kind of fundamental advance is possible only through basic research, which thrives only in an atmosphere of scientific freedom of investigation. It takes decades to destroy research capital and potential of a nation, but this is precisely the effect of socialization of medicine. The only countries that have been nationalized long enough to see the full effect on research of a controlled medical system are Germany, Austria, and the Soviet Union.

Germany and Austria had a golden era of medical research between 1850 and 1910 unequalled in any other country. During that period, no fewer than 280 internationally famous German and Austrian medical scientists emerged. In the 60 years since 1910, fewer than 30 great names have appeared. Twelve Nobel Prizes in Medicine and Physiology have been awarded to Germans and Austrians since 1910; of those, only 4 were won by physicians, and 3 of these were awarded for work done before 1910. Arguments that two world wars destroyed science in Europe are clearly not valid. Following the wars there was a great resurgence in other sciences: chemistry, physics, mathematics, biochemistry, photography, optical-instrument design, and engineering. From 1910 until the present Germans and Austrians have won 20 Nobel Prizes in chemistry and 12 in physics. Of all the sciences, medicine suffered the greatest eclipse, and it is now apparent that the eclipse will not soon end. This occurred in the countries that pioneered in plans for socializing medicine, starting with Bismarck's original plan in Germany. "For some strange reason, the Bismarck milieu either failed to attract genius, or, having attracted some managed to stifle it."

In Russian medicine, as in all other aspects of Russian life, unquestioning adherence to official and orthodox thought has been encouraged since 1917. To all physicians around the world, the names of Betz, Eck, Korsakoff, Metchnikov, and Pavlov are familiar as a few of the many Russians who have contributed important advances to medical research. All of these men made their contributions before 1917. Since the Revolution and the socialization of medicine that accompanied it, there have been only two important contributions by Russians: corneal grafting in 1931 and virologic research by Zdanov. The Russians have discovered one antibiotic: gramicidin. It has no clinical usefulness.

Most other Western European countries have nationalized

medicine too recently to have felt the effects of the death by slow strangulation that is inevitable. Britain has felt an increasing squeeze from lack of research talent in the 24 years of the NHS, because of both the restrictive financial support of the government and the loss of some of its best physicians by emigration. It should come as no surprise that the center of medical research in the world today is in the country that has resisted socialization the longest, the United States.

"You can't get a doctor when you need one." This is a commonly heard complaint and is usually followed by some suggestion that controlling the medical profession will correct all that and assure availability of treatment for all people at all times. The facts strongly suggest that any form of nationalization will not significantly alter the current pattern of distribution of physicians and availability of facilities.

The Soviet Union has had as great a problem as other countries in providing reasonable distribution of physicians, despite the most highly controlled and organized medical system in the world. Fifty years after socialization, the ratio of doctor to population in the world of the Soviet Union was 1:375. At the same time, the ratio in the United States was 1:633. Although there are almost twice as many physicians in the Soviet Union and despite compulsory assignment of physicians to rural areas, "in smaller cities there is one doctor for each 4,300 citizens; in some of the more remote autonomous republics and districts there may be as many as 5,000 to 8,000 persons for every physician." This compares to the ratio of one physician for every 2,145 citizens in rural areas of the United States. It is argued that the Russian deficiencies in distribution are compensated by the use of more paramedical personnel. In fact, the ratio of physicians to other health personnel in Russia in 1970 was 1:3, whereas the comparable ratio in the United States in 1970 was 1:10. If there is a shortage of health-care personnel in this country, it is no greater than and perhaps less than the shortage in the Soviet Union, which for 50 years has had the sort of coercive control of health-care planning that many in this country are seeking for us.

At the close of the Second World War, the British hospital system was in disarray; many facilities had been bombed, and, because of the financial demands of the war, hospital practice and facilities were behind other Western countries by about 10 years.

The passage of the NHS in 1948 had the effect of locking the hospitals into an already outmoded system. Yet, during the first 20 years of the NHS, not a single new general hospital was built in Britain. The director of the NHS during that period admits that this was a grave error and gives as the reason that he, holding nearly absolute power over the system, had simply chosen other priorities for spending the government's money—namely, preventive medicine and mental health. Under a coercive system, people are not free to select their own priorities by choosing how to spend their money; so artificial needs are created and satisfied while the real ones go unanswered.

Let us look now at a few vital statistics. Does government control of the health industry actually improve the health statistics of a nation? There is no evidence that it does, but there is considerable evidence that the health indices are far more closely related to social and economic factors than systems of medical care. The only statistics supporting the notion of superior health care under collectivist systems has been that of infant mortality. The United States, we are told, ranks only twelfth to eighteenth in the world in infant mortality. What we are not told is that infant mortality means different things in different countries; statistical methods vary from country to country and even within countries (e.g., the United States); there are no standard criteria for determining infant mortality; even if there were standard criteria, countries with a population of small average stature have infants of small size and therefore an artificially lower infant mortality; reporting of births is the responsibility of parents in some countries; reporting of deaths is not rigidly enforced in others; legalized abortions in some countries have an unknown effect on lowering infant mortality; and there are known to be racial differences in deaths of infants.

If the United States is to be compared to another nation, it should be one of about equal population, spread out over an entire continent, and of multiethnic origin. Such a country is the Soviet Union. In the United States, with its emphasis on free enterprise in medical care and with a chaotic nonsystem, the infant mortality in 1970 was 19.7 per 1,000 births. In Russia, in the same year, following a 60-year tradition of state-controlled medicine with a heavy emphasis on public health and preventive medicine, the infant mortality rate was 26.0, an increase of 30 percent over ours. Whatever benefits we get from nationalization of the health system, improved health will not be one of them.

In this presentation I have dealt with some popular misconceptions. I have shown that health care is, in fact, not a right. I have shown that political implementation of that nonright has not improved the health of people; it has only consolidated the political power of those in public office or seeking office. I have not discussed other misconceptions, such as the headline-seeking charges that there is a "crisis" in American medical care, that doctors and inefficient management are primarily responsible for the rising cost of health care, that there is an objectively meaningful shortage of doctors, or that government-managed health care will be less expensive than free-enterprise health care. None of these commonly heard statements is true.

I have presented this material with three points of view and with three different motives. First, and most important, I speak as a citizen with a profound interest in regaining the freedom, zest for life, and sense of the nobility of man that have been part of the United States since its founding and in preserving true human rights for myself, my children, and anyone else who agrees that they're worth saving. Second, I speak as a physician who recognizes as his first and highest professional obligation the welfare of his patients and who demands the right to fulfill his freely chosen obligation to his patients by the uncoerced exercise of his own best judgment in his patients' interest. Third, I speak as a potential patient who knows that the real victims of nationalization of medicine are the patients themselves, and who wants the kind of medical care available to him that can be offered only by professionals who are not beholden to anyone but their patients.

Affirmative Response

Hildegarde Peplau

When I was a child it was common practice in neighborhoods of the economically deprived to repeat this quatrain:

> This is a free country,
> Free without a doubt;
> If you haven't had your supper
> You are free to go without.

Today, in this country and indeed all around the world, there are millions of children and adults who are free to go without food, education, and health care. In contrast, there are millions of people who enjoy unprecedented affluence and who therefore experience their freedom in the context of all the advantages of life, liberty, and the pursuit of happiness that money can buy.

Two generations ago, before television and COMSAT, this contrast in the quality of lives of the rich and the poor could go unnoticed. Today, modern technology and communications systems have helped to inform the "have nots" about the quality of life of those who are affluent. As a consequence, a rising tide of

Revised from an article in *Image* 7 (February 1974): 4-10.

expectations and demands for opportunities for a better life for all people is becoming the most important social issue of our time.

The two rights recognized most recently in this country—civil rights and the right to health care—grew out of the emerging act of contemporary civilization. The scope and speed of the implementation of these rights in the decades ahead will indeed be a measure of the extent of man's humanity to man. What is a right? How do rights evolve? How are they implemented and safeguarded? Such questions will be discussed in this subchapter in relation to the right to health care.

Webster defines a right as "that to which one has a just claim: any power vested in a person by the law, custom, etc."[1] Furthermore, ethical considerations determine those rights that are warranted on a moral basis. A right, then, is a social invention, an idea that arises from among the people, an expectation or demand formulated as a claim, which then attains further power through custom or law.

The code of ethics of the nursing profession has two principles that, by giving the moral approval of the profession as a whole to belief in and implementation of the right to health care,[2] commit nurses as follows: (1) the "nurse provides services with respect for the dignity of man, unrestricted by considerations of nationality, race, creed, color, or status" and (2) the "nurse works with members of health professions and other citizens in promoting efforts to meet health needs of the public."

The interpretive statements of the second principle are instructive, for they imply the nursing profession's belief in the right of all people to health care:

> It is increasingly recognized that society's need and mounting demand for comprehensive health services can be met only through a broad and intensive effort on the part of both the community and the health professions. The nurse . . . has an obligation to participate actively and responsibly in professional, interprofessional, and community endeavors designed to meet the health needs of the public.[3]

There are various kinds of rights and, because rights are inventions that arise out of changing social needs and beliefs, their nature changes. Some rights persist; others do not. For example, not much credence is given to the idea of "divine rights," a concept once thought to embody just claims by mortals that were granted by God. Such rights were held by sovereigns who presided over monarchies, a form of government that is rare today. Earlier in the history of humankind—and even today in remote, primitive societies—property was held in common by the group. Over the years, communal rights were superceded in many societies by property rights and laws to safeguard them. Property rights evolved after individual ownership of property had become customary, and disputes were settled by formulation and promulgation of a new form of the right concerning property. In Massachusetts, John Wise—using data from a 1672 study by Pufendorf—eloquently attempted to persuade people to become aware of the inadequacies inherent in the principles underlying then-existing forms of government such as monarchies, aristocracies, and oligarchies. The theory of natural rights, which Wise promoted, became one of the important roots of our democratic philosophy and form of government. Wise's instinctive sympathy for the lot of the common people helped him to generate the moral fervor for his leadership in persuading an acceptance of natural rights. The same subject was debated in the 1600s in England:

> Out of the debates around the camp fires of the army had come a new philosophy that rested on the principles that the individual, both as Christian and citizen, derives from nature certain inalienable rights which every church and every state is bound to respect. This far-reaching doctrine of natural rights, to the formulation of which many thinkers had contributed and which received later its classic form from the pen of Locke, was the suggestive contribution of Puritanism to political theory with the aid of which later liberals were to carry forward the struggle.[4]

The lesson is clear: New principles and new social practices are generated when thoughtful people confront new circumstances and seek new ways to deal with them. This was the case when the constitutional principle of individual freedom was established. The right to determine one's own belief, the right to join freely with others to express that belief, and safeguards for the exercise of that right are all aspects of the principle.[5] The Bill of Rights—which guarantees such inalienable rights as life, liberty, and the pursuit of happiness—is a kind of promissory note which says that the individual has and cannot surrender these rights; laws and social custom, however, provide the means to claim them.

The right to health care is implied by the Bill of Rights, for without health—or at least the opportunity to attain or sustain it—the rights to life, liberty, and the pursuit of happiness become relatively meaningless because hunger, ignorance, pain, illness, and disease are more compelling coercions.

The right to health care derives from a rapidly growing social awareness of a degree or kind of inequality in our society. The public is beginning to realize that those who are affluent and know how to locate available resources, get health care of the highest quality, whereas the "have nots" and the uninformed get little care, no care, or low-quality care.

This social awareness is not unlike that which led to the Civil Rights Act of 1954. A majority of the citizenry noticed, or were forced to recognize, gross inequalities and inequities in the treatment of Blacks as compared to whites in this society. More importantly, they were willing to formulate their belief in equal treatment for all as a right and do something about it. The need to grant such new rights and implement them through laws and social practices was eloquently stated by Paine:[6]

> Every age and generation must be free to act for itself in all cases as the ages and generations which preceded it. The vanity and presumption of governing beyond the grave is the most ridiculous and insolent of all tyrannies. . . . Every generation is, and must be, competent to all of the purposes which its occasions require. It is the living, and not the dead, that are to be accommodated.

It is the social conscience of a people—however it is awakened—that, generation after generation, determines what new rights are to be granted, the provisions to be made in order to safeguard and implement each new right, and the punishments to be meted out when such rights are violated. By establishing a right, society takes on a moral obligation; granting a right signals an expansion of the human heart and mind. The right to health care is based on a facet of love: It signifies that human beings value one another or, to use Fromm's definition of love, that they care as much for others as for themselves.[7]

There is ever-increasing evidence that the world community as well as American society believes in the principle of health care as a right. According to the report of the President's Commission on Human Rights:

> The concept of health as a human right in the United States has evolved slowly but steadily throughout our history. It is reflected first in the passage near the end of the 18th century of an act for the relief of sick and disabled seamen. This national action was largely a self-protective measure on behalf of port cities that were burdened by the cost of sick nonresident seamen. Further measures followed, including quarantine to protect against importation of disease from other countries and the spread of epidemic disease domestically.
>
> In the early part of the 20th century, state and local public health departments were organized to protect the population of their jurisdiction through control of infectious diseases and environmental sanitation. Although there was some expansion of their role during the first 35 years of this century, they remained confined, except for contagious diseases, to the preventive aspects of health. There was no national health program except for seamen, military personnel, foreign quarantine, and the interstate aspects of the control of the spread of epidemic diseases between states. Gradually, however, provision was made for providing directly, or assisting individuals in the purchase of, medical care. This occurred first in local general public assistance programs and, subsequently, in State-administered and Federally assisted programs for indigent aged, the blind, dependent children, and crippled children.
>
> Health as a human right has meaning only when health is understood to be a state of complete physical, mental, and social well-being and not merely the absence of disease or infirmity. This was recognized in national legislation in the United States for the first time in the Partnership for Health Act of 1966. This basic concept of the right to health as embodied in this legislation may be stated in terms of four goals as follows:
>
> 1. Every person should have maximum protection against diseases that need not happen and against illness and injury resulting from the hazards of the modern environment.
> 2. Every person should have ready access to basic medical care—despite social, economic, geographic, or other barriers—and should have the assurance of continuity of quality service through diagnosis, treatment and rehabilitation.

3. Every person should also have maximum opportunity for developing his capabilities in an environment that is not merely safe but conducive to productive living.
4. All activities conducted in pursuit of health should be carried out with full attention to the dignity and integrity of the individual.

There is a long road to travel from the recognition of a human right in law and in the mind of man to its attainment. Only the first step on this journey is now being taken.[8]

The United Nations Universal Declaration of Human Rights, adopted by the General Assembly in 1948, also states the right to health care. This document was endorsed in 1971 by the International Council of Nurses and in 1972 by the American Nurses' Association. The constitution of the World Health Organization states: "The enjoyment of the highest attainable standard of health is one of the fundamental rights of every human being."

In 1969 the American Medical Association House of Delegates passed a resolution stating that it is "the basic right of every citizen to have available to him adequate health care." The Ulman Bill, which established the National Health Corps, holds that "health care is an inherent right." The 1972 platform of the Democratic Party stated, "We endorse the principle that good health is a right of all Americans," whereas the Republican Party held that "Our goal is to enable every American to secure quality health care at reasonable cost." Lyndon B. Johnson was quoted in a *New York Times* article as follows:

Over all the years of our nation's existence, we have been setting goals for ourselves and striving tirelessly to meet them. These goals have been both slogans and the substance of national affairs for generation after generation: Full employment. Decent wages. Adequate housing. Education for everyone. Opportunity for all. Good health, good medical care, good hospitals for even the least among us.[9]

A right is a social convention. It is an ideal shared by a significant number of citizens in a community, state, nation, or the world and a goal to which they aspire. A consensus concerning such beliefs is the basis for a commitment to their implementation. A right is a claim that individuals can make on the community; the community, by agreeing to that claim, becomes obligated to ensure availability and access to whatever social practices or services the right requires. Thus a right is a common good, a benefit that cuts both ways—for the individual and collectively. In this sense, a right is a social commitment that all or most citizens make to each other for their mutual benefit. As with all beliefs, there is never 100 percent concurrence, and so there is always the risk that some persons will not honor the right but instead will deceive, disrupt, and otherwise fail to yield to claims on the right. Laws and the courts provide mechanisms to arbitrate such disputes and confirm or deny the intended meaning of a principle such as a right.[10] Laws "put teeth" into a right in order to safeguard it by prescribing penalties for its denial. Each individual must exercise his claim to a right: "It is possible to establish a right and still acknowledge the importance of the individual's duty to exercise that right subject to reasonable conditions."[11]

Rights also obligate society as a whole to provide through its political, financial, and educational systems those "reasonable conditions" in which availability and access to the required social practices or services can be ensured. When changes in attitudes are involved, political, professional, and other social leaders are expected to use their powers of leadership and persuasion to guide the public in the acceptance of an established right and its implementation or to use orderly debate and reasonable discussion to change it.

From the foregoing discussion it is possible to identify the steps in the evolution of a right and its introduction into the mainstream of society:

1. Citizens become aware of new needs or an inequality, and discussions about it generate consensus around an ideal.
2. The ideal is identified, formulated, and stated as a right.
3. Further social agreement and widespread acceptance of the stated right are obtained.
4. The right is implemented by (a) changing attitudes through leadership, persuasion, etc.; (b) establishing the practices and services required and making them available; and (c) establishing safeguards against denial of the right.

5. Individuals claim the right by availing themselves of its implementing practices.
6. Evidence of the good of the community deriving from implementation of the right become observable.

Although adequate documentation has been given for acceptance of the idea that health care is a right, further exploration of why it should be accepted may aid discussion. Some of the reasons lie deep in human history; others are contemporary. Certain Biblical injunctions are still sound guidelines: for example, Jesus said, "Whatever ye have done to the least of these ye have done it unto me." One may also cite an affirmative answer to the question, "Am I my brother's keeper?" Furthermore, the social belief in freedom is relatively meaningless when health concerns cannot be met. An important contemporary reason is a matter of social conscience: How can those of us whose basic needs are met every day close their eyes to the plight of those whose basic needs are not being met, whose growth as human beings is hampered, whose capacities are never fully realized, and whose existence is marginal and forever marred by vulnerability to ill health? No one individual can rectify this situation; only the national and worldwide communities—by pooling their resources—can hope to hold out an opportunity for healthy development and healthy living for all people. To state that health care is a right is to work steadily toward providing that opportunity.

Our country has the wealth; once the right has been stated, the public is more likely to set its priorities in terms of the ideal. In implementing the right to health care, we become people who care enough to want each human being, despite "the slings and arrows of outrageous fortune," to have the opportunity to reach for healthy living with community health.

If the United States can spend billions of dollars on a senseless war, it can surely afford a kidney dialysis machine for everyone who needs it; it can surely provide the expensive treatment required for every hemophiliac; it can surely provide schools for its mentally retarded, health care for its aging citizens, and treatment for its deviants. When implemented fully, the health-care right will lead us toward a society in which there are no rejects from the human services that provide opportunities for healthy living.

Although it may be difficult to comprehend a new form of society in which the only rejects are self-selected, many recent discussions about wiping out poverty suggest this possibility. Evidence has been presented to show that there already exists substantial and growing public agreement, national and world-wide, that health care is a right. Moral reasons for implementing this right have been suggested. The urgent remaining questions are the following: (1) How broadly should *health* be defined? (2) How should the health right be further implemented? (3) How should denial of the right be handled?

DEFINING HEALTH AND HEALTH CARE

All the goals cited by Lyndon Johnson (see above) he described as "simple and basic," and all of them have to do with health—particularly if the WHO definition is accepted. This definition holds that "health is not merely the absence of disease but includes a sense of well-being." According to this concept, *health* is a broad term that includes all of the external and internal conditions and processes conducive to a "state of complete physical, mental, and social well-being and not merely the absence of disease or infirmity." There is growing pressure to broaden the definition of *health*. Citizens, consumer advocates, and health-right groups are stressing the deleterious effects on health of air and water pollution, unsafe mines and buildings, as well as cars and many other industrial products.[12] More pressure is being put on government regulatory agencies already established to safe-guard the health of the public through their functions of surveil-lance of food and drugs. Parents of the mentally retarded are demanding schools, not hospitals, to ensure the full development of their child's potential. Moreover, the explosion of scientific knowledge relevant to a broad concept of health suggests the need to use many different disciplines in view of the impossibility of any one profession's mastering and applying such knowledge.

What is emerging is the concept that *health care is more than medical care*; it is an interdisciplinary enterprise requiring the integration of knowledge from many sources and the interrelation-ship of many different independent professions. This requirement is implicit in the Health Manpower statistics, which show that there are over 3 million health-care personnel in traditional facilities and that 330,000 of these are physicians.

But the controversy over the definition of health care—that is, the problem of extending the definition beyond the medical model and beyond the unilateral purview and control of medicine—is broader than the matter of knowledge and numbers. The controversy is most glaring in the field of mental health, where the medical model since the 19th century has been used to conceptualize and treat mental illness in the same mode as physical illness. In the last decade or so there has emerged a growing literature that rejects this model, viewing it as an impediment to the development of innovative, nonmedical corrective practices for all but those few clients who have clearly medically related problems such as brain disease. An expanding group of professionals and social scientists is pointing out the harmful effects of diagnostic labeling, hospitalization, and prescribed-drug abuse of persons whose behavior is regarded as deviant. An increasing number of these clients and former patients have established new institutions based on their own concepts of health for the purposes of solving their own health problems—such as drug addiction, alcoholism, and mental illness. In 1971 the state of Pennsylvania established for the mentally retarded "the right to education," thereby shifting to nonmedical agencies the responsibility for meeting broadly defined health needs of these citizens.

The process of redefining health care as more than medical care is likely to go on for years, but one consequence will be a clarification of the concept of health as a basis for full implementation of the health-care right.

IMPLEMENTATION OF THE HEALTH-CARE RIGHT

Implementation has already begun. Every congressional bill signed into law by the President that has to do with education of health personnel, provision of health services, or support for the health of individuals is an implementation of the right to health. Federal financing of medical education and nursing education, the Mental Health Act of 1946, the Social Security Act, Medicare, and Medicaid are all examples, and there are others too numerous to mention. The government has even financed "planning for planning for health care." Finally, a majority of the public and 51 percent of all physicians agree that there should be national health insurance. The issues now include what form it should take, what should be included as coverage, who should be the carrier, and whether the poor will have patient-care health services of the same high quality as the rich. All of these efforts are directed toward implementation of the right to health. There are also tests in the courts, through class-action suits, to determine, for example, whether the loss of constitutional rights implicit in involuntary commitment of mental patients implies a court-guaranteed right to treatment.

Of course, not all health care is provided by professionals. There is an increasing interest in self-help, as indicated by the exhibits—there was even a gadget to lift sagging facial muscles and thus eliminate the need for plastic surgery—and the attendance at a recent health fair at the New York Coliseum. The public media, television, radio, newspapers, and journals, are all helping to slowly close the gap between available scientific knowledge and what laymen know about the health of themselves and their communities. As indicated earlier many lay-oriented groups are forming for the purpose of helping members with health-related problems. The heavy use of over-the-counter drugs and vitamins, as well as the interest in "organic" foods and health-related exercises and recreation, are all attempts by the lay population to sustain health and to exercise the health right by individual means.

HANDLING THE DENIAL OF RIGHTS

Except for the laws already enacted and health regulations already in effect, this aspect of the right is not yet well developed. As Bazelon put it: "When important rights, such as the right to treatment, are at stake, courts must become involved whether they are ill-informed or well-informed . . . courts have a long history of participating in disputes of the most technical and esoteric sort."[13] When professionals fail to honor the health-care right to treatment, the right to know the consequences of research, the right to know what is involved (e.g., the risks of surgery), etc., a dispute arises between professionals and consumers. As these disputes are settled, new guidelines and principles are established. One current question has to do with the accountability of professionals: unless all health professionals, separately and interprofessionally, resolve this matter, this aspect of the health-care right will also be settled in the public domain.

REFERENCES: AFFIRMATIVE RESPONSE

1. *Webster's Collegiate Dictionary*, 5th ed.; "right."
2. "Code for Nurses with Interpretive Statements," American Nurses' Association, 1956.
3. Ibid.
4. Vernon Louis Parrington, *Main Currents in American Thought* (New York: Harcourt, Brace, 1930, part I), p. 10.
5. Ibid.
6. Op Cit., Part I, p. 335.
7. Erich Fromm
8. "For Free Men in a Free World: A Survey of Human Rights in the United States," Department of State Publication 8434, July 1969, pp. 166-68.
9. *New York Times*, 21 September 1972, p. 47.
10. Gary Saretsky and James Mecklengurger: "See You in Court," *Saturday Review*, 14 October 1972, pp. 50, 55-56.
11. Boijon Jaeger, "Government and Hospitals: A Perspective on Health Politics," *Hospital Administrator* 17, no. 1, p. 49.
12. Stanley Klein, "A Product-Injury Surveillance System," *Saturday Review,* 23 September 1972, pp. 67-8.
13. David I. Bazelon, "The Right to Treatment: The Courts' Role," *Hospital and Community Psychiatry* 20, no. 5 (May 1969): 19.

BIBLIOGRAPHY: IS HEALTH CARE A RIGHT?

Peplau, Hildegarde. "Is Health Care a Right?—Affirmative Response." *Image* 7 (February 1974): 4-10.
Sade, Robert M. "Medical Care as a Right: A Refutation." *New England Journal of Medicine* 283, no. 2(December 1972): 1288
————. "National Health Insurance: Rx for Disease." *Reason*, September 1974, pp. 4-9.
————. "What About Health Care for the Poor?" *Private Practice*, October 1974, pp. 24-31.
————. "Is Health Care a Right?—Negative Response," *Image* 7 (February 1974): 11-19.

UNIT IV

Traditional Views of
Health and Illness

The chapters in this unit will enable the reader to:

1. Develop a level of awareness of the background and health problems of ethnic people of color.
2. Understand some traditional beliefs of ethnic people of color with respect to health and illness.
3. Understand the traditional pathways to health care and the relationship between these pathways and the American health-care system.
4. Understand certain manpower problems of each of the communities discussed.
5. Be more familiar with the available literature regarding each of these communities.

The following exercises are appropriate to all chapters in Unit IV:

1. Familiarize yourself with some literature of the ethnic community of color. That is, read literature, poetry, or a biography of a member of each of these communities. (See Bibliographies for Chapters 9, 10, 11, and 12.)
2. Familiarize yourself with the history and sociopolitical background of each of these communities.

The questions that follow should be thoughtfully considered.

3. What are the traditional definitions of health and illness in each of these communities?
4. What are the traditional methods of maintaining health?
5. What are the traditional ways of preventing illness?
6. What are the traditional ways of treating an illness?
7. What are traditionally thought to be the causes of an illness?
8. Who are the traditional healers? What functions do they perform?

The final unit of this book explores the traditional beliefs about health and illness, as well as the practices and current health-care problems of ethnic people of color. The ethnic people of color of the United States are the Asian Americans, the Black Americans, the Native-American Indians, and the Hispanic Americans. According to the 1970 census the population of the United States was 203,212,912. Whites comprised 87.64 percent of the population (178,107,190 people). The ethnic/racial minorities constituted 16.82 percent of the population (34,178,324 people). There is general agreement that these latter census data are incorrect: it is believed that the greatest numbers of uncounted people exist within the groups under discussion.

The following charts and comments are included as introductory material to provide the reader with a brief overview of the demographic and economic backgrounds of ethnic people of color.

The *Asian-American population*, according to the 1970 census, was 1,522,106. According to some sources, this figure is an underenumeration because some Asian Americans were not clearly identified in the census. Of the listed number, 65,510 were Korean; 336,731 Filipinos; 431,583 Chinese; 588,324 Japanese; and 99,958 Hawaiians. The greater percentage of this population (61.3 percent) falls between the ages of 18 and 64, whereas 31.6 percent is under 18 years of age and 7.1 percent is 65 years of age or over. Educational levels for members of the population over 25 years of age are as follows: 26 percent of the population completed 0 to 8 years of school; 41.0 percent, 9 to 12 years; 12.6 percent, 13 to 15 years; and 20.4 percent 16 or more years.

In 1969 the national mean size of Asian-American families below the poverty line in the United States was 3.8 members. There were 26,545 poverty families, and since the total number of Asian-American families was 300,164, 8.8 percent of all families fell below the poverty line. Of the total population, 10.9 percent were persons in families that fell below the poverty level. The mean family income in 1969 was $12,420, and the per capita income was $5,415. In 1970, 8.8 percent of the households had a female head. The percentage of households that had more than one person per room was 17.2 percent.

The *Black-American population,* according to the 1970 census, was 25,105,722. The National Urban League cites this figure as

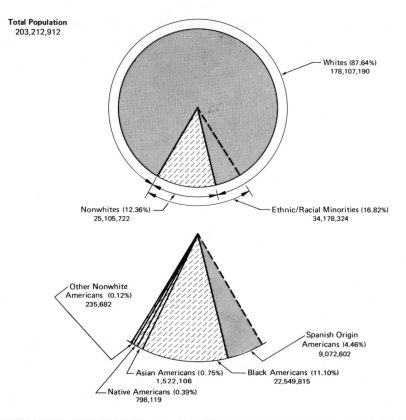

Total Population
203,212,912

Whites (87.64%)
178,107,190

Nonwhites (12.36%)
25,105,722

Ethnic/Racial Minorities (16.82%)
34,178,324

Other Nonwhite
Americans (0.12%)
235,682

Spanish Origin
Americans (4.46%)
9,072,602

Asian Americans (0.75%)
1,522,106

Black Americans (11.10%)
22,549,815

Native Americans (0.39%)
798,119

CHART 1   Ethnic/racial minorities, U.S. population, 1970 census. There is general agreement that census data are understatements of population enumeration and that the net undercount is a greater proportion of nonwhites than of whites (estimated 9.5% and 2.2%, respectively, in 1960). The National Urban League cites a 1970 net underenumeration for the Black population of 1.873 million. In its 1971 fiscal year report, the Cabinet Committee on Opportunities for Spanish-Speaking People estimates that 12 million persons in the United States are of Spanish-speaking background. Some Native-American experts believe the 1970 figure for Indians is an undercount of at least 500,000. Some Asian Americans are not clearly identified in census data. There is also considerable disagreement over the terminology and criteria used in classification and presentation of racial/ethnic data, particularly the definition of "white" and "nonwhite" as race/color descriptors. For a more comprehensive consideration of these issues, see (1) H.S. Shryock and J.S. Siegel, "Racial and Ethnic Composition" *The Methods and Materials of Demography,* 2nd printing (rev.), 2 vols. (Washington, D.C.: U.S. Government Printing Office, 1973, chap 9, pp. 252-81; (2) Commission on Civil Rights, *To Know or Not to Know* (Washington, D.C.: U.S. Government Printing Office, 1973.) (Courtesy of American Public Health Association.)

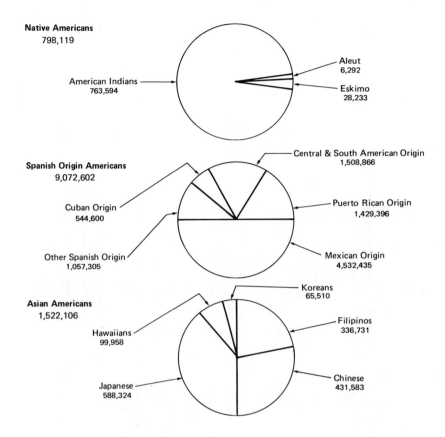

Native Americans
798,119

American Indians
763,594

Aleut
6,292

Eskimo
28,233

Spanish Origin Americans
9,072,602

Central & South American Origin
1,508,866

Cuban Origin
544,600

Puerto Rican Origin
1,429,396

Other Spanish Origin
1,057,305

Mexican Origin
4,532,435

Asian Americans
1,522,106

Koreans
65,510

Hawaiians
99,958

Filipinos
336,731

Japanese
588,324

Chinese
431,583

CHART 2   Minority population composition, 1970 U.S. census. Data from U.S. Department of Commerce, Bureau of the Census, U.S. Government Printing Office, Washington, D.C. (1) American Indians 1970, PC(2)-1F, June 1973, p. x. (2) Persons of Spanish Origin 1970, PC(2)-1C, June 1973, p. ix. (Courtesy of American Public Health Association.)

a net underenumeration for the Black population of at least 1.873 million people. The greatest number of these nonwhites falls between the ages of 18 and 64 years (50.7 percent), whereas 42.3 percent of the particular population is under 18 years and 7.0 percent is 65 years and older. Educational levels for members of this nonwhite population over 25 years are as follows: 43.8 percent of the population has completed 0 to 8 years of school; 45.9 percent, 9 to 12 years; 5.9 percent, 13 to 15 years; and 4.4 percent, 16 or more years.

In 1969 the national mean size of Black families below the

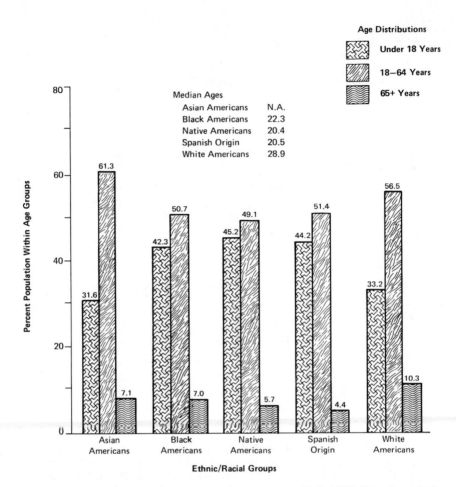

CHART 3   Age distributions, ethnic/racial groups, U.S. 1970. Data from U.S. Department of Commerce, Bureau of the Census, U.S. Government Printing Office, Washington, D.C. (1) Japanese, Chinese, Filipinos in the U.S. 1970, PC(2)-1G, July 1973, pp. 2, 61, and 120; (2) Negro Population 1970, PC(2)-1B, May 1973, p. 2; (3) American Indians 1970, PC(2)-1F, June 1973, p. 1; (4) Persons of Spanish Origin 1970, PC(2)-1C, June 1973, p. 1; (5) U.S. Summary, Detailed Characteristics 1970, PC(1)-D-1, February 1973, pp. 591-592. (Courtesy of American Public Health Association.)

poverty line in the United States was 4.7 members; there were 1,454,586 families below the poverty level.   Of a total of 4,863,401 Black families, 29.9 percent were below the poverty level.   The mean family income was $7,074 and the per-capita income was $3,557.   The mean earning level for Black males was

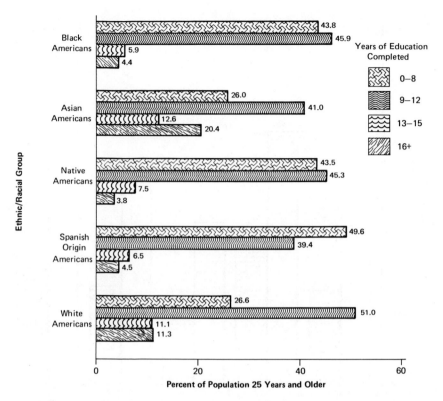

CHART 4   Years of school completed for individuals 25 years of age and older. Data from U.S. Department of Commerce, Bureau of the Census, U.S. Government Printing Office, Washington, D.C. (1) Japanese, Chinese, Filipinos in the U.S. 1970, PC(2)-1G, July 1973, pp. 9, 68, 130; (2) Negro Population 1970, PC(2)-1B, May 1973, p. 20; (3) American Indians 1970, PC(2)-1F, June 1973, p. 26; (4) Persons of Spanish Origin 1970, PC(2)-1C, June 1973, p. 56; (5) U.S. Summary, Detailed Characteristics 1970, PC(1)-D-1, February 1973. (Courtesy of American Public Health Association.)

$4,158, and for females it was $2,687. In 1970, the percentage of families with female heads was 27.4, and the percentage of households with more than one person per room was 19.4.

The *Hispanic-American population*, according to the 1970 census, was 9,072,602. However, this figure is also considered to be an underenumeration. In 1971 the Cabinet Committee on Opportunities for Spanish-speaking People estimated that 12 million people are of Spanish-speaking origin in the continental United States. Of this total population, 544,600 people are of

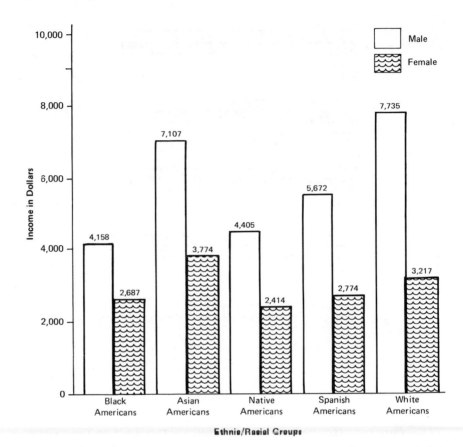

CHART 5 Mean earning levels for population 16 years and over per ethnic/ racial groups, 1969. Data from U.S. Department of Commerce, Bureau of the Census, U.S. Government Printing Office, Washington, D.C. (1) Japanese, Chinese, Filipinos in the U.S. 1970, PC(2)-1G, July 1973, pp. 13, 72, and 131; (2) Negro Population 1970, PC(2)-1B, May 1973, p. 30; (3) American Indians 1970, PC(2)-1F, June 1973, p. 27; (4) Persons of Spanish Origin 1970, PC(2)-1C, June 1973, p. 67; (5) U.S. Summary, Detailed Characteristics 1970, PC(1)-D-1, February 1973. (Courtesy of American Public Health Association.)

Cuban origin; 1,508,866 are of Central and South American origin; 1,429,396 are of Puerto Rican origin; 4,532,435 are of Mexican origin; and 1,522,106 are of other Spanish origin. According to the 1977 census projections, by the mid-1980s people of Spanish origin will comprise the largest single minority in the United States.

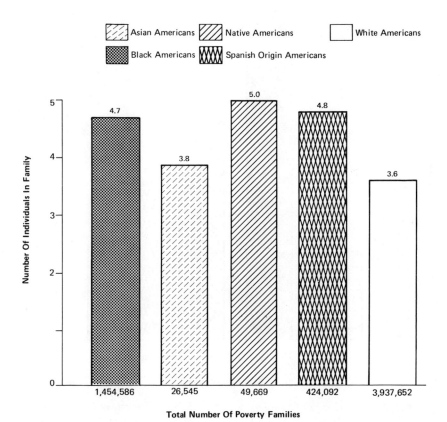

CHART 6   Mean size of families below poverty level by ethnic/racial group, U.S. 1969. Data from U.S. Department of Commerce, Bureau of the Census, U.S. Government Printing Office, Washington, D.C. (1) Japanese, Chinese, Filipinos in the U.S. 1970, PC(2)-1G, July 1973, pp. 43, 101, and 161; (2) Negro Population 1970, PC(2)-1B, May 1973, p. 143; (3) American Indians 1970, PC(2)-1F, June 1973, p. 120; (4) Persons of Spanish Origin 1970, PC(2)-1C, June 1973, p. 121; (5) U.S. Summary, Detailed Characteristics 1970, PC(1)-D-1, February 1973. (Courtesy of American Public Health Association.)

The largest number of people in this population group fall between the ages of 18 and 64 (51.4 percent); 44.2 percent are under the age of 18; and only 4.4 percent are over 65. The overall level of education for individuals 25 and over is as follows: 49.6 percent of the population have completed 0 to 8 years of education; 39.4 percent, grades 9 to 12; 6.5 percent, grades 13 to 15; and 4.5 percent 16 or more years of education.

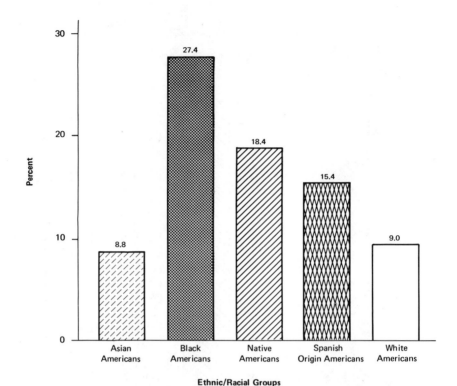

CHART 7   Percentage of families with female heads by ethnic/racial groups, U.S. 1970. Data from U.S. Department of Commerce, Bureau of the Census, U.S. Government Printing Office, Washington, D.C. (1) Japanese, Chinese, Filipinos in the U.S. 1970, PC(2)-1G, July 1973; (2) Negro Population 1970, PC(2)-1B, May 1973; (3) American Indians 1970, PC(2)-1F, June 1973; (4) Persons of Spanish Origin 1970, PC(2)-1C, June 1973; (5) U.S. Summary, Detailed Characteristics 1970 PC(1)-D-1, February 1973. (Courtesy of American Public Health Association.)

In 1969 there were 424,092 families with a mean size of 4.8 who fell below the defined poverty level for that year. There were also 2,004,411 Spanish-origin families below the 1969 poverty level. The mean family income in 1969 was $8,192 and the per capita income was $4,165. In 1969 males earned a mean income of $5,672 and females had a mean income of $2,744. In 1970, 15.4 percent of families had female heads of households, and 25.7 percent of the households had more than one person per room.

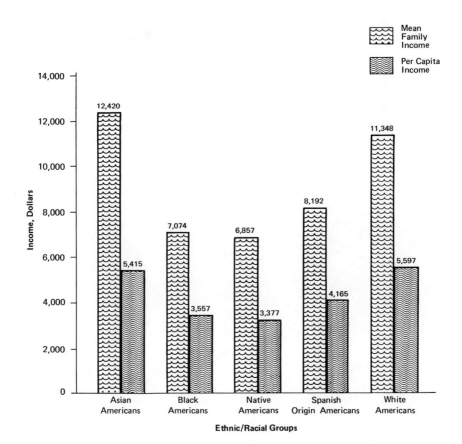

Mean
Family
Income

Per Capita
Income

CHART 8   Mean family income and mean per capita income by ethnic/racial
group, U.S. 1969. Data from U.S. Department of Commerce, Bureau of the
Census, U.S. Government Printing Office, Washington, D.C. (1) Japanese,
Chinese, Filipinos in the U.S. 1970, PC(2)-1G, July 1973, pp. 42, 24; 101,
72; 160, 131; (2) Negro Population 1970, PC(2)-1B, May 1973, pp. 143, 31;
(3) American Indians 1970, PC(2)-1F, June 1973, pp. 120, 61; (4) Persons of
Spanish Origin 1970, PC(2)-1C, June 1973, pp. 121, 67; (5) U.S. Summary,
Detailed Characteristics 1970, PC(1)-D-1, February 1973, pp. 919, 836.
(Courtesy of American Public Health Association.)

The *Native-American population*, according to the 1970 census,
was 798,119.   Of this number, 763,594 are American Indians,
6,292 are Aleut, and 28,233 are Eskimos.   The greatest number of
people (49.1 percent) fall between the ages of 18 and 64 years;
45.2 percent of the population is below 18 years of age; and 5.7
percent of the population is 65 years of age and older.   Schooling
completed by individuals 25 years and older is as follows: 43.5

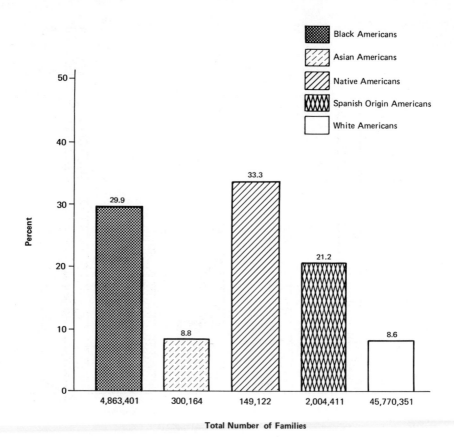

CHART 9   Percentage of families below poverty level by ethnic/racial group, U.S. 1969. Data from U.S. Dept. of Commerce, Bureau of the Census-Special Reports, 1970. U.S. Department of Commerce, Bureau of the Census, U.S. Government Printing Office, Washington, D.C. (1) Japanese, Chinese, Filipinos in the U.S. 1970, PC(2)-1G, July 1973, pp. 42, 101, 160; (2) Negro Population 1970, PC(2)-1B, May 1973, p. 143; (3) American Indians 1970, PC(2)-1F, June 1973, p. 120; (4) Persons of Spanish Origin 1970, PC(2)-1C, June 1973, p. 121; (5) U.S. Summary, Detailed Characteristics 1970, PC(1)-D-1, February 1973, p. 988. (Courtesy of American Public Health Association.)

percent of the population has completed 0 to 8 years; 45.3 percent 9 to 12 years; 7.5 percent 13 to 15 years; and 3.8 percent 16 or more years.

In 1969 the mean family size below the poverty level was 5.0; the total number of families below the poverty level was 49,669.

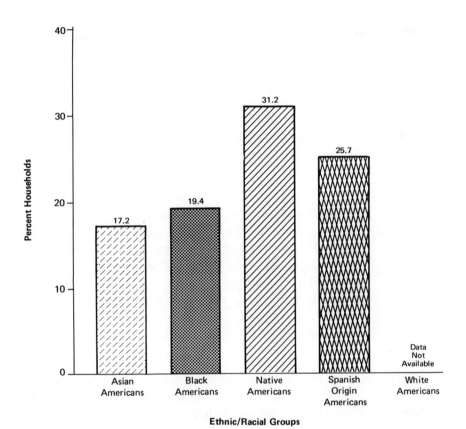

CHART 10   Percentage of households with more than one person per room by ethnic/racial group, 1970. Data from U.S. Department of Commerce, Bureau of the Census, U.S. Government Printing Office, Washington, D.C. (1) Japanese, Chinese, Filipinos in the U.S., 1970, PC(2)-1G; July 1973, pp. 47, 105, 165; (2) Negro Population 1970, PC(2)-1B, May 1973, p. 153; (3) American Indians 1970, PC(2)-1F, June 1973, p. 129; (4) Persons of Spanish Origin 1970, PC(2)-1C, June 1973, p. 136; (5) Information not available for the White population. (Courtesy of American Public Health Association.)

Of the total 149,122 Native-American families, 33.3 percent fell below the poverty level. These figures represent the highest percentage of families below the poverty level for all ethnic or racial groups in the United States in 1969.

In 1969 the mean income for the Native-American family was $6,857. The per capita mean income was $3,377. The mean earning level for the native American male was $4,405, and that for the female was $3,377. These income figures are the lowest for all ethnic or racial groups in the United States at that time.

In 1970, 18.4 percent of these families had female heads. The percentage of households with more than one person per room was 31.2, which means that Native Americans are relegated to the poorest housing in terms of density.

In the discussion of the health and illness beliefs and practices of each ethnic group of people, the following information is included:

> Traditional definitions of health;
> Traditional forms of epidemiologic beliefs;
> Traditional names and symptoms of a given disease;
> Traditional sources of "medical" assistance;
> Traditional remedies;
> Problems the group encounters in dealing with the health-care system;
> The current health-care provider manpower.

It must be kept in mind that this information is general and not universal. It is *not* specific to any one person. However, a given person's personal health care and behavior during illness may well have their roots in the individual's traditional belief system. Thus, if we are caring for a person from one of the ethnic or racial minority groups and we find that there are problems in our interactions or with the patient's compliance, an understanding of traditional beliefs may be helpful. If we understand that these beliefs may well differ from our own, this can help us as well as the consumer to resolve the problems that occur. In addition, the tendency to disrespect a person who does not practice his personal health care as we think he should can be dissipated when we understand the underlying reasons for that individual's unique behavior.

Among all people there is agreement that good health is essential for survival. If we are sick, we cannot work, we cannot provide food for ourselves, and we cannot survive and reproduce. Thus satisfactory health is mandatory for our existence. Yet the definition of health and the means of preserving it vary from people to people. It has already been demonstrated earlier in this book that there is great disagreement among health workers as to what health is. Yet professionals expect other people to accept *their* "nondefinition."

As there are differences in the meaning of health, so are there differences in the meaning of illness. What does illness mean to others? Is it simply the symptoms of a disease, or is it more? What causes illness from a traditional viewpoint? Who are the native, traditional healers, and what methods do they use to treat and heal disorders? How do native healers differ from physicians? What resources are available to a person when he seeks traditional health care?

Research carried out by medical sociologists and anthropologists in the area of health and illness beliefs has been done with the intent to discover and understand these folk ways. There is currently much criticism among ethnic groups who have been studied. They question the meaning of these studies and the interpretations of the researchers. However, despite these criticisms, the work of sociologists and anthropologists is helpful if used as a stepping stone. Thus, in this Unit, the overall results of these studies will be looked at from a specific standpoint. They will be referred to and recommended for further examination in order to *help* health-care providers understand the behaviors and attitudes of the people for whom they care. In addition, I include bibliographic resources that have been recommended by the members of a given community.

It is important to note that much of the literature regarding the health and illness beliefs of any group of people is contradictory. One research report will indicate that a given group of people view health as a reward for good behavior. Another will state that people of the same cultural background believe that health is a matter of chance—something that may be here today, and luck will determine how long it will remain. Yet another study will indicate that some illnesses are believed to be caused by witchcraft, and others by natural elements.

In no way do I wish to imply that (a) any of these findings are universally accurate, or (b) all health care should be based on them. What is important to note about these studies is that they do give, in part, some understanding as to *why* there may be two (or more) conflicting viewpoints between provider and consumer regarding a diagnosis and treatment regimen.

Statements about the health practices of chosen ethnic communities are based not only on the existing literature, as noted, but also on:

1. Data collected from surveys of students, including ethnic students of color, over a 5-year period;
2. Information shared by guest lecturers who are both health-care providers and members of the discussed communities;
3. Data collected from the author's interviews with health-care consumers and providers over a period of 8 years.

CHAPTER 9

Health and Illness in the Asian-American Community

The members of the Asian-American community have their origins in China, Hawaii, the Phillipines, Korea, and Japan. This chapter will focus on the traditional health and illness beliefs and practices of the Chinese Americans, not merely because of space requirements but also because those of the other Asians derive, in part from the Chinese.

BACKGROUND

The Chinese immigration to the United States began over 100 years ago. In 1850, there were only 1,000 Chinese inhabitants in this country; in 1880, there were well over 100,000. This rapid increase in part owed to the discovery of gold in California and in part to the need for cheap labor to build transcontinental railroads: these immigrants were laborers who met the needs of the dominant society. Like many early immigrant groups, they came here intending only to stay as temporary workers. Mainly men came. They clung closely to their customs and beliefs and stayed together in their own communities. The hopes that they had for a better life when they came to the United States did not materialize. Subsequently, many of the workers and their kin returned to China before 1930. Part of the disharmony and disenchantment occurred because these immigrants were not white and did not have the same culture and habits as whites. For these reasons, they were not welcomed, and many jobs were not open to them. For example, Chinese immigrant workers were excluded from many mining, construction, and other hard-labor jobs even though the transcontinental railroad was constructed mainly by numerous Chinese laborers. Between 1880 and 1930, the population declined by nearly 20 percent. Another factor that added to and helped perpetuate this decline in population was a series of exclusion acts that halted further immigration. The people who remained behind were relegated to menial jobs such as cooking and dishwashing. The Chinese workers first took these jobs in the West, and later they moved eastward throughout the United States. They tended to move to cities where they were allowed to let their entrepreneurial talents surface—their main pursuits included running small laundries, food shops, and restaurants.

The people settled in tightly knit groups in urban neighborhoods that took the name "Chinatown." Here they were able to maintain the ancient traditions of their homeland. These individuals were hard workers and, in spite of the dull, menial jobs that were usually available to them, they were able to survive.

Both immigration laws of the United States and political problems in China had an effect on the nature of today's Chinese population. When the exclusion acts were passed, many men were left alone in this country without the possibility of their families joining them. For this reason, a great majority of the men spent many years alone. In addition, the political oppression experienced by the Chinese in the United States was compounded when, at a time immigration laws were relaxed here after World War II, people were unable to return to or leave China because of that country's restrictive new regulations. However, by 1965, a large number of refugees who had relatives here were able to come to this country. These individuals settled in the Chinatowns of America, causing the population of these areas to swell: the rate of increase since 1965 has been 10 percent per year.

One outstanding problem being faced in the nation's Chinatowns is that of elderly men who are sick and alone. Men have always

outnumbered women in Chinatown because, as stated earlier, so
many of them came to the United States without their families
and then were unable to send for them.[1]

TRADITIONAL DEFINITIONS OF HEALTH AND ILLNESS

Chinese medicine teaches that health is a state of spiritual and
physical harmony with nature. In ancient China, the task of the
physician was to prevent illness. A first-class physician was one
who not only cured an illness but could also prevent disease from
occurring. A second-class physician had to wait for his patients to
become ill so that he could then treat them. The physician was
paid by the patient while he was healthy; when illness occurred,
payments stopped. Indeed, the physician not only was not paid
for his services when the patient became ill, but he also had to
provide and pay for the needed medicine.[2]

In order to understand the Chinese philosophy of health and illness, it is necessary to look back at the age-old philosophies from
which more current ideas have evolved. The foundation rests in
the religion and philosophy of Taoism. Taoism originated with a
man named Lao Tzu, who is believed to have been born about
604 B.C. The word *Tao* has several meanings: way, path, or
discourse. On the spiritual level, it is the way of ultimate reality.
It is the way of all nature, the primeval law that regulates all
heavenly and earthly matters. In order for one to live according
to the Tao, one must adapt oneself to the order of nature. Chinese
medical works revere the ancient sages who knew the way and
"led their lives in *Tao*."[3]

The Chinese view the universe as a vast, indivisible entity; each
being has a definite function within it. No one thing can exist
without the existence of the others. Each is linked in a chain
that consists of concepts related to each other in harmonious
balance. Violating this harmony is like hurling chaos, wars, and
catastrophies upon humankind—the end result of which is illness. Individuals must adjust themselves wholly within the environment. Five elements—wood, fire, earth, metal, and water—
constitute the guiding principles of humankind's surroundings.
These elements can both create and destroy each other. For

example: "Wood creates fire," "two pieces of wood rubbed together produce a spark," "wood destroys earth," "the tree sucks strength from the earth." The guiding principles arise from this "correspondences" theory[4] of the cosmos.

In order for a person to remain healthy, his actions must conform to the mobile cycle of the correspondences. The exact directions for achieving this were written in such works as the *Lu Chih Ch'un Ch'iu* (Spring and Autumn Annals) written by Lu Pu Wei, who died circa 230 B.C.

Four thousand years before William Harvey described the circulatory system in 1628, *Huang-ti Nei Ching* (Yellow Emporer's Book of Internal Medicine) was written. This is the first known volume that describes the circulation of blood. It described the oxygen-carrying powers of blood and defined the two basic world principles: *yin* and *yang*, powers that regulate the universe. *Yang* represents the male, positive energy that produces light, warmth, and fullness. *Yin* represents the female, negative energy—the force of darkness, cold, and emptiness. *Yin* and *yang* exert power not only over the universe but also over human beings.

The various parts of the human body correspond to the dualistic principles of *yin* and *yang*. The inside of the body is *yin*; the surface of the body is *yang*. The front part of the body is *yin*; the back is *yang*. The five *ts'ang* viscera—liver, heart, spleen, lungs, and kidney—are *yin*; the six *fu* structures—gallbladder, stomach, large intestine, small intestine, bladder, and "warmer"—are *yang*. (The "warmer" is now believed to be the lymph system.) The diseases of winter and spring are *yin*; those of summer and fall are *yang*. The pulses are controlled by *yin* and *yang*. If *yin* is too strong, the person is nervous and apprehensive and catches colds easily. If the individual does not balance his *yin* and *yang* properly, his life will be short. Half of the *yin* forces will be depleted by age 40, at 50 the body will be sluggish, and at 60 the *yin* will be totally depleted, at which time the body will deteriorate. *Yin* stores the vital strength of life. *Yang* protects the body from outside forces, and it too must be carefully maintained. If *yang* is not cared for, the viscera will be thrown into disorder and circulation will cease. *Yin* and *yang* cannot be injured by evil influences. When *yin* and *yang* are sound, the person is living in peaceful interaction with his mind and body in proper order.[4]

Chinese medicine has a long history. The Emperor Shen Nung,

who died in 2697 B.C., was known as the patron god of agriculture. He was given this title because of the 70 experiments he performed on himself by swallowing a different plant every day and studying the effects. During this period of self-experimentation, Nung discovered many poisonous herbs and rendered them harmless by the use of antidotes, which he also discovered. His patron element was fire, for which he was also known as the Red Emperor. The Emperor Shen Nung was followed by Huang-ti, whose patron element was earth. Huang-ti was known as the Yellow Emperor and ruled from 2697 to 2595 B.C. The greater part of this man's life was devoted to the study of medicine. Many people ascribe to him the recording of the *Nei Ching*, the book that embraces the entire realm of Chinese medical knowledge. The treatments described in the *Nei Ching*—which became characteristic of Chinese medical practice—are almost totally aimed at reestablishing balances that are lost within the body when illness occurs. Disrupted harmonies are regarded as the sole cause of disease. Surgery was rarely resorted to; when it was, it was used primarily to remove malignant tumors. The *Nei Ching* is a dialogue between Huang-ti and his minister, Ch'i Po. It begins with the concept of the Tao and the cosmologic patterns of the universe and goes on to describe the powers of the *yin* and *yang*. This learned treatise discusses in great detail the therapy of the pulses and how a diagnosis can be made on the basis of alterations in the pulse beat. It also describes various kinds of fevers and the use of acupuncture.[5]

The Chinese view their bodies as a gift given to them by their parents and forebearers. A person's body is not his personal property. It must be cared for and well maintained. Confucius taught that "only those shall be truly revered who at the end of their lives will return their physical bodies whole and sound."

The body is composed of five solid organs (*ts'ang*), which collect and store secretions, and five hollow organs (*fu*), which excrete. The heart and liver are regarded as the noble organs. The head is the storage chamber for knowledge, the back is the home of the chest, the loins store the kidneys, the knees store the muscles, and the bones store the marrow.

The Chinese view the functions of the various organs as comparable to the functions of persons in positions of power and responsibility in the government. For example, the heart is the ruler over all the other civil servants, the lungs are the adminis-trators, the liver is the general who initiates all the strategic actions, and the gallbladder is the decision maker.

The organs have a complex relationship that maintains the balance and harmony of the body. Each organ is associated with a color. For example, the heart—which works in accordance with the pulse, controls the kidneys, and harmonizes with bitter flavors—is red. In addition, the organs have what is referred to as an "aura," the meaning of which, in the medical context, is health. The aura is determined by the color of the organ. In the balanced, healthy body, the colors look fresh and shiny.[6]

As stated earlier, disease is caused by an upset in the balance of *yin* and *yang*. However, the weather, too, has an effect on the body's balance and the body's relationship to *yin* and *yang*. For example, heat can be injurious to the heart, and cold is injurious to the lungs. Overexertion is also harmful to the body. Prolonged sitting is harmful to the flesh and spine, and prolonged lying in bed can be harmful to the lungs.

Disease is diagnosed by the Chinese physician through inspec-tion and palpation. During inspection, the Chinese physician looks at the tongue (glossoscopy), listens and smells (osphretics), and asks questions (anamnesis); during palpation, the physician feels the pulses (sphygmopalpation).

The Chinese believe that there are many different pulse types, which are all grouped together and must be felt with the three middle fingers. The pulse is considered the storehouse of the blood, and a person with a strong, regular pulse is considered to be in good health. By the nature of the pulse, the physician is able to determine various illnesses. For example, if the pulse is weak and skips beats, the person may have a cardiac problem. If the pulse is too strong the person's body is distended.[7]

There are six different pulses, three in each hand. Each pulse is specifically related to various organs, and each pulse has its own characteristics. According to ancient Chinese sources, there are 15 ways of characterizing the pulses. Each of these descriptions accurately determines the diagnosis. There are seven *piao* pulses (superficial) and eight *li* pulses (sunken). An example of an illness that manifests with a *piao* pulse is headache; anxiety manifests with a *li* pulse. The pulses also take on a specific nature with various conditions; for example, specific pulses are associated with epilepsy, pregnancy, and the time just before death.[8]

The Chinese physician is also aided in making a diagnosis by the appearance of the patient's tongue. There are more than 100 varieties of conditions that can be determined by glossoscopic examination. The color of the tongue and the part of the tongue that does not appear normal are the essential clues to the diagnosis.[9]

Breast cancer has been known to the Chinese since early times: "The disease begins with a knot in the breast, the size of a bean, and gradually swells to the size of an egg. After seven or eight months it perforates. When it has perforated, it is very difficult to cure."[10]

TRADITIONAL METHODS OF HEALING

Traditional Healers

The physician was the primary healer in Chinese medicine. Physicians who had to treat women encountered numerous difficulties because men were not allowed to touch women directly. Thus a diagnosis might be made through a ribbon that was attached to the woman's wrist. As an alternative to demonstrating areas of pain or discomfort on a woman's body, an alabaster figurine was substituted. The area of pain was then pointed out on the figurine.[11]

Not much is known about women doctors except that they did exist. Women were known to possess a large store of medical talent. There were also midwives and female shamans. The female shamans possessed gifts of prophecy; they danced themselves into ecstatic trances and had a profound effect on the people around them. However, as the knowledge that these women possessed was neither known or understood by the general population, they were feared rather than respected. They were said to know all there was to know about life, death, and birth.[12]

Chinese Pediatrics

Babies are breast fed because neither cows' milk nor goats' milk is acceptable to the Chinese. Sometimes babies are nursed for as long as four or five years.

Since early times the Chinese have known about and practiced immunization against smallpox. A child was innoculated with the live virus from the crust of a pustule from a smallpox victim. The crust was ground into a powder, and this powder was subsequently blown into the nose of the healthy child through the lumen of a small tube. If the child was healthy, he did not generally develop a fullblown case of smallpox but instead acquired immunity to this dreaded disease.[13]

Acupuncture

Acupuncture is an ancient Chinese practice of puncturing the body to cure disease or relieve pain. The body is punctured with special metal needles at points that are precisely predetermined for the treatment of specific symptoms. According to one source, the earliest use of this method was recorded between 106 B.C. and 220 A.D.; however, according to other sources, it was used earlier than this time. This treatment modality stems from diagnostic procedures described earlier. The most important aspect of the practice of acupuncture is the acquired skill and ability to know precisely where to puncture the skin. There are nine needles used in acupuncture, each with a specific purpose. The following is a list of the needles and their purposes:[14]

> Superficial pricking: arrowhead needle
> Massaging: round needle
> Knocking or pressing: blunt needle
> Venous pricking: sharp three-edged needle
> Evacuating pus: swordlike needle
> Rapid pricking: sharp, round needle
> Puncturing thick muscle: sharp, round needle
> Puncturing thick muscle: long needle
> Treating arthritis: large needle
> Most extensively used: filiform needle

The specific points of the body into which the needles are inserted are known as meridians. Acupuncture is based on the concept that certain meridians extend internally throughout the body in a fixed network. There are 365 points on the skin where these lines emerge. As all of the networks merge and have their outlets on the skin, the way to treat internal problems is to puncture the meridians, which are also categorically identified in terms of *yin* and *yang*, as are the diseases. The treatment goal is to restore the balance of *yin* and *yang*.[15] The practice of this art is far too complex to explain in greater detail in these pages; there is a suggested reading list included in the Annotated Bibliography.

Readers may find it interesting to visit acupuncture clinics in their area. After the therapist carefully explains the art and science of acupuncture, one may be able to grasp the fundamental concepts of this ancient treatment. The practice of acupuncture is based in antiquity, yet it took a long time for it to be accepted as a legitimate method of healing by practitioners of the Western medical system. Currently, there are numerous acupuncture clinics that attract a fair number of non-Asians, and acupuncture is being used as a method of anesthesia in some hospitals.

Moxibustion

Moxibustion has been practiced for as long a time as acupuncture. Its purpose, too, is to restore the proper balance of *yin* and *yang*. Moxibustion is based on the therapeutic value of heat, whereas acupuncture is a cold treatment. Thus acupuncture is used mainly in diseases in which there is an excess of *yang*, and moxibustion is used in diseases in which there is an excess of *yin*. Moxibustion is performed by heating pulverized wormwood and applying this concoction directly to the skin over certain specific meridians. Great caution must be used in this application because it cannot be applied to all the meridians that are used for acupuncture. Moxibustion is believed to be most useful during the period of labor and delivery, if applied properly.[16]

There are additional ancient forms of treatment, such as local and widespread body massage and special exercises performed to prolong life.

Herbal Remedies

Medicinal herbs were widely used in the practice of ancient Chinese healing. Many of these herbs are available and in use today.

Herbology is an interesting subject to explore in more detail. The gathering season of an herb was important for its effect. It was believed that some herbs were better if gathered at night and that others were more effective if gathered at dawn. The ancient sages understood quite well the dynamics of growth because it is now known that a plant may not be effective if the dew has been allowed to dry on its leaves.[17] The herbalist believes that the ginseng root can be harvested only at midnight in a full moon if it is to have therapeutic value. Ginseng's therapeutic value is due to its nonspecific action. The herb, which is derived from the root of a plant that resembles a man,* is recommended for use in more than two-dozen ailments including anemia, colics, depression, indigestion, impotence, and rheumatism.[18] It has maintained its reputation for centuries and continues to be a highly valued and widely used substance.

To release all the therapeutic properties of ginseng and to prepare it properly are of paramount importance. Ginseng must not be prepared in anything made of metal because it is believed that some of the necessary constituents are leeched out by the action of the metal. It must be stored in crockery. It is boiled in water until only a sediment remains. This sediment is pressed into a crock and stored. Some of the specific uses of ginseng follow.

> *To stimulate digestion*: Rub ginseng to a powder, mix with the white of an egg, and take three times per day.
> *As a sedative*: Prepare a light broth of ginseng and bamboo leaves.
> *For faintness after childbirth*: Administer a strong brew of ginseng several times a day.
> *As a restorative for frail children*: Give a dash of raw, minced ginseng several times per day.[19]

There are countless Chinese medicinal herbs, but none is so famous as ginseng.

I had the opportunity to visit, with one of my Asian-American students, an import-export store in Boston's Chinatown where they sell Chinese herbs—if one has the proper prescriptions. The front of the store is a gift shop that attracts numerous tourists.

---

*Early Chinese healers believed that if the name of a plant resembled the disease in question, the plant would be effective in the treatment of the disease.

In the back there is a room that is separated from the rest of the store. We were allowed to enter this room when the student explained to the proprietor, in Chinese, that I was her teacher and that she had brought me to the store to purchase herbs. We stayed there for quite a long time, observing the people who came in with prescriptions. The man carefully weighed different herbs, mixed them together, and dispensed them. We asked to purchase some of the herbs that he took from the drawers lining the entire wall behind him. He refused to sell us anything except some of the preparations that were on the counter because a prescription was necessary to purchase any of the herbal compounds that he prepared. Undaunted, we purchased a wide variety of herbs that could be used for indigestion, in addition to ointments and liniments used for sore muscles and sprains.

In addition to herbs and plants, the Chinese used a number of other products with medicinal and healing properties. Some of these products were also used in ancient Europe and are still used today. For example, in China, boys' urine was used to cure lung diseases, soothe inflamed throats, and dissolve blood clots in pregnant women. In Europe it was used during the two World Wars as emergency treatment for open wounds. Urea is still used today as a treatment that promotes the healing of wounds. Other popular Chinese remedies include the following:[20]

> Deer antlers: Used to strengthen bones, increase a man's potency, and dispel nightmares
> Lime calcium: Used to clear excessive mucus
> Quicksilver: Used externally to treat venereal diseases
> Rhinoceros horns: Highly effective when applied to pus boils; an antitoxin for snakebites
> Turtle shells: Used to stimulate weak kidneys and to remove gallstones
> Snake flesh: Eaten as a delicacy to keep eyes healthy and vision clear
> Seahorses: Pulverized and used to treat gout

Current Health Problems

The residents of Chinatowns today experience all the socioeconomic and other problems faced by other groups who are the victims of poverty and poor living conditions. The overall death rates for both men and women are higher than those of their white counterparts. Tuberculosis, although eradicated from the greater population, still leaves its mark on the Chinese, whose living conditions continue to be crowded. It has been reported that many ill and disabled Chinese return to China to die; thus figures may even be low with respect to the overall morbidity and mortality rates.[21]

Poor health is found among the residents of Chinatowns partly because of poor working conditions. Many of the people work long hours in restaurants and laundries and receive the lowest possible wages for their hard work. Many cannot afford even minimal, let alone preventive, health care.[22]

Language difficulties and adherence to native Chinese culture compound problems already associated with poverty, crowding, and poor health. Many people still prefer the traditional forms of Chinese medicine and seek help from Chinatown "physicians" who treat them with traditional herbs and other methods. Often they do not seek help from the Western system at all. Others use Chinese methods in conjunction with Western methods of health care, although the Chinese find many aspects of Western medicine distasteful. For example, they cannot understand why so many diagnostic tests, some of which are painful, are necessary. However, they accept the practice of immunization and the use of x-rays.

They are most upset by the practice of drawing blood. Often, numerous blood tests are done, and the Chinese people cannot understand why they are necessary. Blood is seen as the source of life for the entire body, and they believe that it is not regenerated. The Chinese people also believe that a good physician should be able to make a diagnosis simply by examining a person; consequently, they do not react well to the often-painful procedures used in diagnostic work-ups. Some people—because of their distaste for this kind of procedure—leave the Western system rather than tolerate the pain. As stated earlier, the Chinese have deep respect for their bodies and believe that it is best to die with their bodies intact. For this reason, many people refuse surgery or consent to it only under the most dire circumstances.[23] This reluctance to undergo intrusive surgical procedures has deep implications for those concerned with providing health care to Asian Americans. Even their reluctance to have blood drawn for diagnostic tests may have its roots in the revered teachings of Confucius.

The hospital is an alien place to the Chinese. Not only are the customs and practices strange, but the patients are often isolated from the rest of their people, which enhances the language barrier and feelings of helplessness. Something as basic as food creates another problem. Hospital food is strange and is served in an unfamiliar manner. As noted in an earlier chapter, the typical Chinese patient rarely complains about what bothers him. Often the only indication that there may be a problem is an untouched food tray and the silent withdrawal of a patient. Unfortunately, the silence may be regarded by the nurses as reflecting good, complacent behavior, and the health-care team exerts little energy to go beyond that assumption. The Chinese patient who says little and complies with all treatment is seen as stoic, and there is little awareness that deep problems may underly this "exemplary" behavior. Ignorance on the part of health-care workers may cause the patient a great deal of suffering.

Much action has been taken in recent years to make Western health care more available and appealing to the Chinese. In Boston, for example, there is a health clinic staffed primarily by Chinese-speaking nurses and physicians who work as paid employees and as volunteers. Most of the common health-related pamphlets have been translated into Chinese and are distributed to the patients. Booklets on such topics as breast self-examination and how to quit smoking are available. Since the language spoken in the clinic is Chinese, the problem of interpreters has been eliminated. The care is personal, and the clients are made to feel comfortable. Unnecessary and painful tests are avoided as much as possible. In addition, the clinic, which is open for long hours, provides social services and employment placements and is quite popular with the community. Although it began as a part-time, store front operation, the clinic is now housed in its own building.[24]

Asian-American Health Manpower

In most areas of health manpower, except nursing, there is a fairly significant number of people representing the Asian-American community: 1.5 percent of physicians, 2.2 percent of dentists, and

3.8 percent of optometrists are Asian Americans. In the nursing profession, the percentage is quite low, with only a small number of Asian-American nurses.[25] Today, the individual who desires to be a physician in China has the option of studying either Chinese or Western medicine. If he selects Western medicine, he is also taught a limited amount of Chinese medicine. As Chinese traditional medicine is becoming better recognized and better understood in the United States, more doors are being opened to those who prefer or understand this mode of treatment.

REFERENCES

1. Frederick P. Li et al., "Health Care for the Chinese Community in Boston," *American Journal of Public Health*, (April 1972), pp. 536-537.
2. Felix Mann, *Acupuncture* (New York: Vintage Books, 1972), p. 222.
3. Houston Smith, *The Religions of Man* (New York: Harper, 1958), pp. 175-192.
4. Heinrich Wallnöfer and Anna von Rottauscher, *Chinese Folk Medicine*, trans. Marion Palmedo (New York: American Library, 1972), pp. 12-16; 19-21.
5. Ibid., pp. 26-28.
6. Ibid., pp. 79-81.
7. Ibid., pp. 97-109.
8. Ibid., p. 99.
9. Ibid., p. 109.
10. Ibid., p. 115.
11. Josephine Dolan, *Nursing in Society: A Historical Perspective* (Philadelphia: Saunders, 1973), p. 30.
12. Wallnöfer and Von Rottauscher, op cit.,[4] pp. 39-40.
13. Ibid., p. 119.
14. Ibid., p. 126.
15. Ibid., pp. 127-128.
16. Ibid., pp. 135-138.
17. Ibid., p. 43.
18. Ibid., pp. 42-43.
19. Ibid., pp. 44-47.
20. Ibid., p. 71.
21. Li et al., op cit.,[1] p. 537.
22. Ibid., p. 538.
23. Ibid.
24. Ibid., p. 539.

25. William H. MacBeath et al., "Minority Chart Health Book" (presented at the 102nd Annual Meeting, American Public Health Association, New Orleans, 20-24 October, 1974), pp. 86-89.

BIBLIOGRAPHY: HEALTH AND ILLNESS IN THE ASIAN-AMERICAN COMMUNITY

Leong, Lucille. *Acupuncture: A Layman's View.* New York: Signet, 1974.

> Acupuncture is, above all, preventive medicine, and the patient is treated as a whole—body, mind, and spirit being inseparable. There is a precept that applies to acupuncture as well as to all Chinese healing. The acupuncturist admonishes: "Curing is not so good as preventing, and preventing is not so good as taking care of oneself." Physicians are paid to keep people healthy; when clients fall ill, they stop payment.

Mann, Felix. *Acupuncture: The Ancient Chinese Art of Healing and How it Works Scientifically.* New York: Vintage Books, 1972.

> This general book discusses the theories of acupuncture, the acupuncture points, the meridians, *yin* and *yang*, various diagnostic and therapeutic techniques, and preventive medicine.

Palos, Stephan. *The Chinese Art of Healing.* New York: Herter and Herter, 1971.

> Palos includes a history of the Chinese art of healing; a discussion of man and nature, *yin* and *yang*; and a description of the human body in ancient Chinese thought. The traditional methods of treatment discussed are acupuncture, moxibustion, remedial massage, and physiotherapy.

Shih-Chen, Li. *Chinese Medicinal Herbs.* Translated by F. Porter Smith and G. A. Stuart, San Francisco: Georgetown Press, 1973.

> Containing an alphabetical listing of numerous Chinese herbs, this book discusses the history and use of each herb. It also includes a glossary of terms. Excellent reference.

Wei-Kang, Fu. *The Story of Chinese Acupuncture and Moxibustion.* Peking: Foreign Languages Press, 1975.

> A booklet that vividly and precisely describes ancient Chinese medical techniques, this work also describes today's search in China for breakthroughs in medical science.

Wollnöfer, Heinrich, and Von Rottauscher, Anna. *Chinese Folk Medicine.* New York: American Library, 1972.

> This book discusses many treatments and alleged cures that

were used in China for centuries. It describes the fundamentals of Chinese medicine and evaluates its approach to anatomy, physiology, and pathology.

FURTHER SUGGESTED READING

Books

Academy of Traditional Chinese Medicine. *An Outline of Chinese Acupuncture*. Peking: Foreign Languages Press, 1975.

Burang, Theodore. *The Tibetan Art of Healing*. London: Watkins, 1974.

Dolan, Josephine. *Nursing in Society: A Historical Perspective*. Philadelphia: Saunders, 1973.

Duke, M. *Acupuncture*. New York: Pyramid, 1972.

Kitano, Harry. *Japanese Americans*. Englewood Cliffs, N.J.: Prentice Hall, 1969.

Kleinman, Arthur; Kunstader, Peter; Alexander, E. Russel; and Gale, James L., editors. *Medicine in Chinese Cultures*. Washington, D.C.: Fogarty International Center, 1975.

Kroening, R. J., and Bresler, D. E. *Acupuncture for Management of Facial and Dental Pain*. Beverly Hills: Center for Integral Medicine, 1972.

Kung, S. W. *Chinese in American Life*. Seattle: University of Washington Press, 1962.

Leslie, Charles, editor. *Asian Medical Systems*. Los Angeles and Berkeley: University of California Press, 1976.

Lyman, Stanford M. *Chinese Americans*. New York: Random House, 1974.

Palos, S. *The Chinese Art of Healing*. New York: Herter & Herter, 1971.

Peterson, William. *Japanese Americans*. New York: Random House, 1971.

Porkert, Manfred. *The Theoretical Foundations of Chinese Medicine*. Cambridge: MIT Press, 1974.

Rechung, Rinpoche. *Tibetan Medicine*. Los Angeles and Berkeley: University of California Press, 1973.

Smith, Houston. *The Religions of Man*. New York: Harper, 1958.

Sue, Stanley, and Wagner, Nathaniel. *Asian American: Psychological Perspectives*. Palo Alto, Calif.: Science and Behavioral Books, 1973.

U.S. Bureau of the Census. *The Asian Americans*. Washington, D.C.: U.S. Government Printing Office, 1973.

Veith, Ilza. *The Yellow Emperor's Classic of Internal Medicine*. Los Angeles and Berkeley: University of California Press, 1972.

Numerous books are currently available in the area of Chinese medicine. For further information and a complete list of literature, I suggest writing to China Books and Periodicals, 125 Fifth Avenue, New York, New York 10003

Articles

Armstrong, M. E. "Acupuncture." *American Journal of Nursing* 72 (September 1972): 1582-1588.

Bersi, Robert M. "In Search of Identity: Asians in America." Report of Activities, Asian American Research Project, California State College, Dominquez Hills, 1971.

Campbell, Teresa, and Chang, Betty. "Health Care of the Chinese in America." *Nursing Outlook* 21 (April 1973): 245-249.

Chung, Hyo Jin. "Understanding the Oriental Maternity Patient." *Nursing Clinics of North America* 12 (March 1977): 67-75.

Kim, Bok-Him C. "Asian Americans: No Model Minority." *Social Work* (May 1973): 44-53.

Li, Frederick P.; Schlief, Nyuk Yoong; Chang, Caroline J.; and Gaw, Albert G. "Health Care for the Chinese Community in Boston." *American Journal of Public Health* 62 (April 1972): 536-539.

Tao-Kim-Hai, Andre M. "Orientals are Stoic." In *Social Interaction and Patient Care*. Edited by James K. Skipper, Jr., and Robert C. Leonard. Philadelphia: Lippincott, 1965, pp. 143-153.

CHAPTER 10

Health and Illness in the Black-American Community

Members of the Black community have their origins in Africa; the majority were brought here as slaves from the west coast of Africa.[1] The largest importation of slaves occurred during the 17th century. Today, there are a number of Blacks who have immigrated to the United States voluntarily—from African countries, the West Indian Islands, the Dominican Republic, Haiti, and Jamaica. However, the vast majority of the people in this community are the descendants of slaves.

BACKGROUND

According to some sources the first Black people to enter this country arrived a year earlier than the Pilgrims, in 1619; other sources claim that Blacks arrived with Columbus in the 15th century.[1] In any event, the first Blacks who came to the North American continent did not come as slaves. However, between 1619 and 1860 more than 4 million people were transported here

The author especially acknowledges those students who, over several years, have provided much of the data for this chapter.

to be indentured as slaves. One need only read a sampling of the many accounts of slavery to appreciate the tremendous hardships that the captured and enslaved people experienced during that time. Not only was the daily life of the slave very difficult, but the experience of being captured, shackled, and transported in steerage was a devastating experience. Many of those captured in Africa died before they arrived here. According to reliable accounts, the strongest and healthiest people were snatched from their homes by slave dealers and transported *en masse* in the holds of ships to the North American continent. In general, the people were not cared for, nor were they recognized as human beings and treated accordingly. Once here, they were sold and placed on plantations and in homes all over the country—it was only later that the practice was confined to the South. Families were separated; children were wrenched from their parents and sold to other buyers. Some slave owners engaged in breeding: men were purchased to serve as breeders, and women were judged as to whether they should be mated with a particular man.[2] Yet, in the midst of all this inhuman and inhumane treatment, the Black family grew and survived. Gutman[3] traces the history of the Black family from 1750 to 1925. His careful documentation of plantation and family records points out the existence of families and family or kinship ties before and after the Civil War, dispelling many of the myths about the Black family and its structure. Despite overwhelming hardships and enforced separations, the people managed in most circumstances to maintain both a family and community awareness.

Ostensibly, the Civil War ended slavery, but in many ways, it did not emancipate Blacks. Daily life after the war was fraught with tremendous difficulty, and Black people—according to custom—were stripped of their civil rights. In the South the people were overtly segregated, and most lived in conditions of extreme hardship and poverty. Those who migrated to the North over the years were subject to all the problems of fragmented urban life: poverty, racism, and covert segregation.[4]

The purpose of these introductory remarks is not to present a detailed study of the life of Black people in this country; pertinent material is cited in the Bibliography. The historic problems of the Black-American community need to be appreciated by the health-care provider who wants to juxtapose modern practices in the context of some of the traditional health and illness beliefs.

TRADITIONAL DEFINITIONS OF HEALTH AND ILLNESS

The traditional definition of health stems from the African belief about life and the nature of being. To the African, life was a process rather than a state. The nature of a person was viewed in terms of energy force rather than matter. All things, whether living or dead, were believed to influence each other. Therefore, one had the power to influence one's destiny and that of others through the use of *behavior*, whether proper or otherwise, as well as through *knowledge* of the person and the world. When one possessed health, one was in harmony with nature; illness was a state of disharmony. Traditional Black belief regarding health did not separate the mind, body, and spirit.[5]

Disharmony—therefore, illness—was attributed to a number of sources, primarily demons and evil spirits. These spirits were generally believed to act on their own accord, and the goal of treatment was to remove them from the body of the ill person. Several methods were employed to attain this result in addition to voodoo, which is discussed in a separate section. The traditional healers, usually women, possessed extensive knowledge regarding the use of herbs and roots in the treatment of illness. Apparently, an early form of smallpox immunization was used by slaves. Women practiced inoculation by scraping a piece of cowpox crust into a place on a child's arm. These children appeared to have a far lower incidence of smallpox than those who did not receive the immunization.

The old and the young were cared for by all members of the community. The elderly were held in high esteem, because the people believed that the living of a long life indicated that a person had the opportunity to acquire much wisdom and knowledge. Death was described as the passing from one realm of life to another[6] —or as a passage from the evils of this world to another state. The funeral was often celebrated as a joyous occasion, with a party after the burial. Children were passed over the body of the deceased so that the dead person could carry any potential illness of the child away with him.

Many of the preventive and treatment practices have their roots in Africa, but have been merged with the approaches of Native Americans to whom the Blacks were exposed and of the whites among whom they lived and served. Thus, then as today, illness was treated in a combination of ways. Methods found to be most useful were handed down through the generations.

TRADITIONAL METHODS OF HEALING

Voodoo

Voodoo involves a belief system often alluded to but rarely described in any detail. At various times, patients may mention terms such as "fix," "hex," or "spell." It is not clear whether voodoo is *fully* practiced today, but there is some evidence in the literature that there are people who still believe and practice it to some extent.[7] It has also been reported that many people continue to fear voodoo and believe that when they become ill they have been "fixed." There are two forms of magic involved: white magic is described as harmless, whereas black magic is quite dangerous. Belief in magic is, of course, ancient.[8]

Voodoo came to this country well over 200 years ago—about 1724, with the arrival of slaves from the West African coast.[9] The people who brought it with them were "snake worshippers." They were initially sold in the West Indies. *Vodu*, the name of their god, became with the passage of time voodoo, an all-embracing term that included the god, the sect, the members of the sect, the priests and priestesses, the rites and practices, and the teaching.*

The sect spread rapidly from the West Indies. In 1782 the governor of Louisiana prohibited the importation of slaves from Martinique because of their practice in voodooism. (Despite the fact that gatherings of slaves were forbidden in Louisiana, small groups practiced voodoo.) In 1803 Blacks were finally allowed to come to Louisiana from the West Indies, and with them came a strong influence of voodoo.[11] The practice entailed a large number of rituals and procedures. The ceremonies were held with large numbers of people, usually at night and in the open country. "Sacrifice and the drinking of blood were integral parts of all the voodoo ceremonies."[12] There were those who believed that this blood was from children; however, it was most commonly thought to be the blood of a cat or young goat. Such behavior evolved from primi-

*Another common term derived from *Vodu* is hoodoo.[10]

tive African rites, to which Christian rituals[13] were added to form the ceremonies that exist today. Leaders of the voodoo sect tended to be women, and stories abound in New Orleans about the workings of the sect and the women who ruled it—such as Marie Laveau.

In 1850, the practice of voodoo reached its height in New Orleans.[14] At that time the beliefs and practices of voodoo were closely related to beliefs about health and illness. For example, many illnesses were attributed to a "fix" that was placed on one person out of anger. *Gris-gris*, the symbols of voodoo, were used to prevent illness or to give illness to others. Some examples of commonly used *gris-gris*[15] follow.

1. Good *gris-gris*. Powders and oils that are highly and pleasantly scented. The following are examples of good *gris-gris*: love powder, colored and scented with perfume; love oil, olive oil to which gardenia perfume has been added; luck water, ordinary water that is purchased in many shades (red is for success in love, yellow for success in money matters, blue for protection and friends).
2. Bad *gris-gris*. Oils and powders that have a vile odor. The following are examples of bad *gris-gris*: anger powder, war powder, and moving powder, which are composed of soil, gunpowder, and black pepper, respectively.
3. Flying devil oil is olive oil that has red coloring and cayenne pepper added to it.
4. Black cat oil is machine oil.

In addition to these oils and powders, a wide variety of colored candles is used, the color of the candle symbolizing the intention. For example, white symbolizes peace; red, victory; pink, love; yellow, driving off enemies; brown, attracting money; and black, doing evil work and bringing bad luck.[16]

There are also a number of Catholic saints or relics to whom or which the practitioners of voodoo attribute special powers. Hence there may be a prominent display of portraits of St. Michael, who makes possible the conquest of enemies; St. Anthony de Padua, who brings luck; St. Mary Magdalene, who is popular with women who are in love; the Virgin Mary, whose presence in the home prevents illness; and the Sacred Heart of Jesus, which cures organic illness.[17] These *gris-gris* are available today and can be purchased in stores in many American cities.

Other Practices

Many Blacks believe in the power of a given individual to heal and help others, and there are many reports of numerous healers among the communities. This reliance on healers reflects the deep religious faith of the people. (Maya Angelou vividly describes this phenomenon in her book, *I Know Why The Caged Bird Sings.*[18]) For example, many Blacks followed the Pentecostal movement long before its present popularity; similarly, people often went to tent meetings and had an all-consuming belief in the healing powers of religion.

There is another practice that takes on significance when one appreciates its historical background: the eating of Argo starch. "Geophagy," or eating clay and dirt, occured among the slaves, who brought the practice to this country from Africa. In *Roots,* Haley mentions that pregnant women were given clay because it was believed to be beneficial to both the mother and the unborn child.[19] In fact, this clay was rich in iron. When clay was not available, dirt was substituted. In more modern times, when people were no longer living on farms and no longer had access to clay and dirt, Argo starch became the substitute.[20]

> It was my fortune, or misfortune to be born into a family that practiced geophagy (earth eating) and pica (eating Argo laundry starch). Even before I became pregnant I showed an interest in eating starch. It was sweet and dry, and I could take it or leave it. After I became pregnant, I found I wanted not only starch, but bread, grits, and potatoes. I found I craved starchy substances. I stuck to starchy substances and dropped the Argo because it made me feel sluggish and heavy.*

It is believed that anemia gave rise to this practice and that in all probability the habit was both the cause and consequence of

*This experience was reported by a student, who consented that her description be included here.

anemia. Clay was eaten by people who were anemic, and the more of it that was eaten, the greater the anemia and greater the craving. The practice or the habit of eating Argo starch today is a substitute for clay ingestion in the past.

CURRENT HEALTH PRACTICES

In the following paragraphs practices employed first to prevent illness and then to treat various types of maladies are described. They do not encompass all of the types of care given to and by the members of the Black community, but they do present a sample of the richness of the folk medicine that has survived over the years.

Prevention

Essentially, health is maintained with the proper diet—that is, eating three nutritious meals a day including a hot breakfast. Rest and a clean environment are also important. Laxatives were and are used to keep the system "running" or "open."

Asafetida—rotten flesh that looks like a dried-out sponge— is worn around the neck to prevent the contraction of contagious diseases. Cod liver oil is taken to prevent colds. A sulfur-and-molasses preparation is used in the spring because it is believed that at the start of a new season people are more susceptible to illness. This preparation is rubbed up and down the back; it is not taken internally. A physician is not routinely consulted and he is not generally regarded as the person to whom one goes for the prevention of disease.

Copper or silver bracelets may be worn around the wrist from the time a woman is a baby or young child. These bracelets are believed to protect the wearer as she grows. If for any reason these bracelets are removed, harm will befall the owner. In addition to granting protection, these bracelets indicate when the wearer is about to become ill: the skin around the bracelet turns black, and she can then take precaution against the impending illness. These precautions consist of getting extra rest, praying more frequently, and eating a more nutritious diet.

Treatment of Illness

The most common and frequently cited method of treating illness is prayer. The laying on of hands is described quite frequently. Rooting, a practice derived from voodo, is also mentioned. In rooting, a person (usually a woman) is consulted as to the source of a given illness, and she then prescribes the appropriate treatment. Magic rituals are often employed.

The following home remedies have been reported by people as being successful in the treatment of disease.

1. Sugar and turpentine are mixed together and taken by mouth to get rid of worms. This combination can be also used to cure a backache when rubbed on the skin from the navel to the back.

2. Numerous types of poultices are employed to fight infection and inflammation. The poultices are placed on the part of the body that is painful and/or infected, in order to draw out the cause of the affliction.

   One type of poultice is made of potatoes. The potatoes are sliced or grated and placed in a bag, which is placed on the affected area of the body. The potatoes turn black and, as this occurs, the disease goes away. It is now believed that, as these potatoes spoil, they produce a penicillin mould that is able to destroy the infectious organism. Another type of poultice is prepared from cornmeal and peach leaves that are cooked together and placed either in a bag or in a piece of flannel cloth. The cornmeal ferments and combines with an enzyme in the peach leaves. The antiseptic from the fermented cornmeal and the enzyme destroy the bacteria and hasten the healing process. A third poultice, made with onions, is used to heal infections and a flaxseed poultice is used to treat earaches.

3. Herbs from the woods are used in a multitude

of ways. Herb teas are prepared—for example, from goldenrod root—to treat pain and reduce fevers. Sassafras tea is frequently used to treat colds. Other herbs that are boiled to make a tea include the root or weed of rabbit tobacco.

4. Bluestone, a mineral found in the ground, is used as medicine for open wounds. The stone is crushed into a powder and sprinkled on the affected area. It prevents inflammation and is also used to treat poison ivy.

5. To treat a "crick" in the neck, two pieces of silverware are crossed over the painful area in the form of an X.

6. Nine drops of turpentine nine days after intercourse act as a contraceptive.

7. Cuts and wounds can be treated with sour or spoiled milk that is placed on stale bread, wrapped in a cloth, and placed on the wound.

8. Salt and pork (salt pork) placed on a rag can also be used to treat cuts and wounds.

9. A sprained ankle can be treated by placing clay in a dark leaf and wrapping it around the ankle.

10. A method for treating colds is with hot lemon water with honey.

11. When congestion is present in the chest and the person is coughing, he can be wrapped with warm flannel after his chest is rubbed with hot camphorated oil.

12. An expectorant for colds consists of chopped raw garlic, chopped onion, fresh parsley, and a little water, all mixed in a blender.

13. Hot toddies are used to treat colds and congestion. These drinks consist of hot tea with honey, lemon, peppermint, and a dash of brandy or whatever alcoholic beverage the person likes and is available. Vicks Vaporub is also swallowed.

14. A fever can be broken by placing raw onions on the feet and wrapping them in warm blankets.

15. Boils are treated by cracking a raw egg, and

peeling the white skin off the inside of the shell, and placing it on the boil. This brings the boil to a head.

16. Garlic can be placed on the ill person or in the room to remove the "evil spirits" that have caused the illness.

THE BLACK MUSLIMS*

Many members of the Black community are practicing Muslims. Religious beliefs are an important part of the Muslim life-style, and health-care providers should be familiar with them. Dietary restrictions consist of eating a strictly kosher diet, and a newly admitted patient who refuses to eat should be asked if he prefers to observe this diet. "Kosher" means that a practicing Muslim does not eat pork or any pork products (such as nonbeef hamburger and ham), or any "soul foods" (such as black-eyed beans, kidney beans, hamhocks, bacon, and pork chops). Muslims consider such foods to be filthy, and they are taught that a "person is what he eats."

Certain foods affect the way a person thinks and acts; therefore, one's diet should consist of food that has a clean, positive effect. Beans—such as black-eyed, kidney, and lima—are avoided because they are hard to digest and are meant for animal (not human) consumption. Muslims do not drink alcohol because they feel that it dulls the senses and causes illness.

Muslims fast for a 30-day period during September and October, at which time they consume no land meat and eat only one meal per day, in the evening. Nothing is taken by mouth from 5 A.M. until sundown, although an ill Muslim is exempt from this rule.

The Muslim life-style is strictly regulated. According to those who have practiced the religion for many generations, this stems in part from the need for self-discipline, which many Black people have not had because of living conditions associated with urban decay and family disintegration. Muslims believe in self-help and

*This material is adapted from a paper prepared by a student who is a practicing Muslim, and who wanted to share her beliefs. She concluded: "I hope this will help a bit in understanding a Muslim who may be a patient."

assist in uplifting each other. The Muslim life-style is not so rigid that the people do not have good times. Good times, however, are tempered with the realization that too much indulgence in sport and play can present problems.

Muslims differ from Seventh Day Adventists and Jehovah's Witnesses. Seventh Day Adventists do not eat pork but do permit smoking and drinking. Jehovah's Witnesses do not believe in using another person's blood—that is, in accepting transfusions. To Muslims, however, life is precious: if they need a transfusion to live, they will accept it. Another fact of hospital life that is important to understand is the refusal of a Muslim who is diabetic to take insulin that has a pork base. If the insulin is manufactured from the pancreas of a pig it is considered unclean and will not be used.

There are many Muslim subsects that differ in practice and philosophy. The members of some sects dress in distinctive clothing—for example, the women wear long skirts and a covering on the head at all times. Other sects are less strict about dress. Moreover, some adherents do not follow the kosher diet and are allowed to smoke and drink alcoholic beverages in moderation. In some sects men practice polygamy and have a number of concubines.

Comments

In the Black community, folk medicine previously practiced in Africa is still employed. The methods have been tried and tested and they are still relied upon. When the people go to a healer or practice voodoo, no class or status distinctions are made. Whoever receives folk treatment is dealt with fairly and honestly. The people have faith in the practices of the healer and in other methods because they work for them and because they believe in them. In fact, the home remedies that are used by some members of the Black community have been employed for many generations. Another reason for their ongoing use is that hospitals are far away from the people who live in rural areas: "By the time you would get to the hospital you would be dead." Yet many of the people who continue to use these remedies live in urban areas in close proximity to hospitals—sometimes world-renowned hospitals.

Nonetheless, the use of folk medicine persists, and many people avoid the local hospital except in extreme emergencies.

Current Health Problems

To the Black person, receiving health care is all too often a degrading and humiliating experience. In many settings, he continues to be viewed as someone beneath the white health-care giver. Quite often the insults are subtle and not "seen" but rather are *experienced* by the Black person. The insult may be intentional or unintentional. An intentional insult is, of course, an *open* remark or mistreatment. An unintentional insult is more difficult to define. A health-care provider may not *intend* to demean a person, yet his action or his tone of voice may be interpreted as insulting. Or the provider may have some underlying fears or difficulties in relating to Blacks that are covert, but the patient quite often senses the difficulty. An unintentional insult may occur because the provider is not fully aware of the client's background and is unable to comprehend many of the client's beliefs and practices. The client, for example, may be afraid of the procedures that he must undergo and the possibility of misdiagnosis or mistreatment. It is not a secret among the people of the Black community that those who receive care in public clinics and hospitals—and even in clinics of private institutions—are the "material" on whom students practice and learn and on whom medical research is done.

A disease that is the major killer among Blacks is hypertension. Compared with the incidence among whites, it is twice as prevalent and kills 3 to 12 times as many people (depending on the age brackets under consideration). It occurs 7 times more often in women of any age group and 15 times more in men between the ages of 15 and 40. Only 20 percent of the people afflicted with hypertension receive adequate treatment.[21] Stress is believed to be the major contributing factor. Other health problems among members of the Black population are substance abuse—that is, drug and alcohol abuse; mental-health difficulties, with a reluctance to seek help; and high maternal and infant death rates. In some parts of the country the incidence is up to 7 times the maternal and infant death rates of the white population. Malnutrition is also a serious problem.[22]

Some Blacks fear or resent health clinics for many reasons. When they have a clinic appointment they usually lose a day's work because they have to be at the clinic at an early hour and often spend many hours waiting to be seen by a physician. They often receive inadequate care, are told what their problem is in medical jargon that they cannot understand, and are not given an identity—being seen rather as a body segment ("the appendix in treatment room A"). Such people experience a tremendous feeling of powerlessness, and feel alienated by the system. In some parts of the country segregation and racism are overt. There continue to be reports of hospitals that refuse admission to Black patients. In one case, a Black woman in labor was not admitted to a hospital because she had not "paid the bill from the last baby." There was not enough time to get her to another hospital, and she was forced to deliver in an ambulance. In light of this type of treatment, it is small wonder that people prefer to use time-tested home remedies rather than be exposed to the humiliating experiences of hospitalization. Another reason for the ongoing use of home remedies is poverty. Indigent people cannot afford the high costs of American health care. Quite often—even with the help of Medicaid and Medicare—the "hidden costs" of acquiring health services, such as transportation and/or child care, are a heavy burden to people and their families. As a result, Blacks may stay away from clinics or out-patient departments, or receive their care with passivity while appearing to be evasive. Some Black patients believe that they are being talked down to by health-care providers and that the providers fail to listen to them. Consequently, they choose to "suffer in silence." White health-care providers know far too little about how to care for a Black person's skin, how to care for his hair, or how to understand both his nonverbal and verbal behavior. Many of the problems that Blacks relate in terms of dealing with the health-care system are universal. However, the inherent racism within the health system cannot be denied. Currently, numerous efforts are being made to overcome these barriers.

Since the 1960s, the health-care services available to Blacks and other people of color have improved. There has been a growing number of community health centers, and the emphasis of health care within these centers has been on health maintenance and promotion. Community residents serve on the boards.

Many services are provided. For example, efforts are made to discover children with high blood levels of lead in order to provide early diagnosis of and treatment for lead poisoning. Once a child is found to have lead poisoning, the law requires that the source of the lead be found and eradicated. Today, apartments cannot be rented to families with young children unless they are free of lead paint. Apartments that are found to have lead paint must be stripped and repainted with nonlead paint. Another ongoing effort by the community health centers is to inform Blacks who are at risk of producing children with sickle cell anemia that they are carriers of this genetic disease. This latter program is fraught with conflict because many people prefer not to be screened for the sickle-cell trait because they fear becoming labeled once the tendency is discovered.

Birth control is another problem that is recognized with mixed emotions. To some, especially women who want to space children or do not want to have numerous children, birth control is a welcome development. People who believe in birth control prefer the idea of selecting the time when they will have children, how many children they will have, and when they will stop having children. To many other people birth control is considered a form of "Black genocide" and a way of limiting the growth of the community. Health workers in the Black community must be aware of both sides of the issue and, if asked to make a decision, remain neutral. The decision must be made by the clients themselves.

As stated earlier in this book, the majority of the members of the health-care profession are, when they enter the profession, steeped in a middle-class value system. In clinical settings such as were just described, these people are being helped to become familiar with and to understand the value systems of other ethnic groups. For example, they are being taught to recognize the signs and symptoms of illness in Blacks and to provide proper skin and hair care. The following are several guidelines that a health-care provider can follow in caring for members of the Black community.

> 1. The education of an ever-increasing number of Blacks in the health professions must continue to be encouraged. Many Black men and women are currently students in schools of nursing as well as in medical schools, social-work programs, dentistry, and other allied health fields.

2. The needs of the patient must be realistically assessed.
3. When a treatment or special diet is prescribed, every attempt must be made to ascertain whether it is consistent with the patient's physical needs, cultural background, income, and religious practices.
4. The patient's belief in and practice of folk medicine must be respected; he must not be criticized for these beliefs. Every effort should be made to assist the patient to combine folk treatment with standard Western treatment as long as the two are not antagonistic. Most people who have a strong belief in folk remedies will continue to use them with or without medical sanctions.
5. Providers should be familiar with formal and informal sources of help in the Black community. The former sources consist of churches, social clubs, and community groups. The latter includes those women who provide care for members of their community in an informal way.
6. The beliefs and values of the health-care provider should not be forced upon the client.
7. The treatment plan and the reasons for a given treatment must be shared with the patient.

REFERENCES

1. Bonnie Bullough and Vern L. Bullough, *Poverty, Ethnic Identity and Health Care* (New York: Appleton, 1972), 41.
2. Alex Haley, *Roots* (New York: Doubleday, 1976).
3. Herbert G. Gutman, *The Black Family in Slavery and Freedom, 1750-1925* (New York: Pantheon, 1976).
4. Bullough and Bullough, op cit.,[1] p. 43; John F. Kain, *Race and Poverty* (Englewood Cliffs, N.J.: Prentice-Hall, 1969), pp. 1-30.
5. Gladys Jacques, "Cultural Health Traditions; A Black Perspective," in *Providing Safe Nursing Care for Ethnic People of Color*, edited by Marie Branch and Phyllis Perry Paxton (New York: Appleton, 1976), p. 116.
6. Ibid., p. 117.

7. Ronald Wintrob, "Hexes, Roots, Snake Eggs? M.D. vs. Occults," *Medical Opinion* 1, no. 7 (1972): 54-61.

8. Langston Hughes and Arna Bontemps, *The Book of Negro Folklore* (New York: Dodd, Mead, 1958), pp. 184-185.

9. Robert Tallant, *Voodoo in New Orleans*, 7th printing (New York: Collier, 1974), p. 19.

10. Ibid.

11. Ibid., p. 21.

12. Ibid., p. 25.

13. Ibid., p. 38.

14. Ibid., p. 73.

15. Ibid., p. 226.

16. Ibid.

17. Ibid., p. 228.

18. Maya Angelou, *I Know Why the Caged Bird Sings* (New York: Bantam, 1969).

19. Haley, op cit.,[2] p. 32.

20. Beverly Dunstin, "Pica during Pregnancy," in *Current Concepts in Clinical Nursing* (St. Louis: Mosby, 1969), Chapter 26.

21. Lauranne Sams, "Blacks and Health Care: Spanning the Life Cycle" (presented at the New England Regional Black Nurses Association, Inc., Meeting, Statler Hilton Hotel, Boston, Mass., 20 May 1977).

22. Ibid.

BIBLIOGRAPHY: HEALTH AND ILLNESS IN THE BLACK COMMUNITY

Angelou, Maya. *I Know Why the Caged Bird Sings.* New York: Random House, 1970.

Maya Angelou confronts her life with wonder and dignity. She tells of her childhood and growth, describes her friends and neighbors, and shows how life flourishes even in the midst of death.

Bennett, John. *The Doctor to the Dead: Grotesque Legends and Folk Tales of Old Charleston.* Westport, Conn.: Negro University Press, 1943.

Contents are folk stories that have been compiled after many years of searching for the various parts of each story.

Grier, William H., and Cobbs, Price M. *Black Rage.* New York: Bantam Books, 1968.

Two Black psychiatrists tell what it is like to be Black in white America. They display the anger, pain, and frustration that is so much a part of a Black person's life.

Griffin, John Howard. *Black Like Me.* Boston: Houghton Mifflin, 1960.

This popular book answers the question: What is it like to be
Black? It is the story of men who destroy other men for
reasons that they do not understand.

Gutman, Herbert G. *The Black Family in Slavery and Freedom, 1750-1925.*
New York: Pantheon Books, 1976.

This work is a study of the Afro-American family between
1750 and 1925. It also discusses the origins and early development of Afro-American culture.

Haley, Alex. *Roots.* Garden City, N.Y.: Doubleday, 1976.

Haley traces his family back to its believed origins in Africa.
It is an intriguing study of the capture of the Black person,
slavery, and emancipation.

Hughes, Langston, and Bontemps, Arna. *The Book of Negro Folklore.* New
York: Dodd, Mead, 1958.

In this book the reader will encounter numerous short folk
tales relating to animals; memories of slavery; God, human
beings, and the devil; black magic and chance; ghosts; and
spirituals.

Osofsky, Gilbert. *Harlem: The Making of a Ghetto.* New York: Harper, 1963.

Osofsky explores the history of the Black community in New
York City. The book describes Black life in New York before
Harlem, and the changes that have occurred in that community.

Parsons, Elsie Clews. *Folk-Lore of the Sea Islands, South Carolina.* Chicago:
Afro-American Press, 1969.

This book is composed of tales, riddles, beliefs, and odds and
ends of Sea Island folk lore. The Sea Islands stretch out along
the coast of South Carolina from Savannah to Charleston,
and the inhabitants are predominately Black. Many of these
folk-lore tales and riddles come from the Bahamas. They
are written in dialect and convey much spirit.

Smith, Lillian. *Killers of the Dream.* Garden City, N.Y.: Doubleday, 1963.

Smith describes the changes of life in the South. She recreates
the texture of the Southern experience and what it is like to
grow up there from infancy to adulthood. She attempts to
show how during this period negative feelings toward Blacks
are allowed to grow.

Tallant, Robert. *Voodoo in New Orleans.* New York: Collier, 1946.

Tallant traces the history of voodoo from its origins in Africa
to its time of greatest popularity in New Orleans. He reports
the legends as they have been passed on through generations,
and describes the dances and *gris-gris* of voodoo.

FURTHER SUGGESTED READINGS

Books

Banks, James A., and Crambs, D. Leah. *Black Self Concept.* New York: McGraw-Hill, 1972.

Clift, Virgil A., editor. *Negro Education in America.* New York: Harper, 1962.

Comer, James P., and Poussaint, Alvin F. *Black Child Care: How to Bring Up a Healthy Black Child in America.* New York: Simon and Schuster, 1975.

Hill, R. *The Strengths of Black Families.* New York: Emerson Hall, 1971.

Luckcraft, Dorothy. *Black Awareness: Implications for Black Patient Care.* New York: American Journal of Nursing Company, 1976.

Malcolm X. *The Autobiography of Malcolm X.* New York: Grove Press, 1964.

Scanzoni, J. *The Black Family in Modern Society.* Boston: Allyn and Bacon, 1971.

Styron, William. *The Confessions of Nat Turner.* New York: Random House, 1966.

Williams, Richard, *The Textbook of Black Related Diseases.* New York: McGraw-Hill, 1975.

Williams, Robert. *Ebonics: The True Language of Black Folks.* St. Louis: The Institute of Black Studies, 1975.

Wright, Richard. *Black Boy.* New York: Harper, 1937.

————. *Native Son.* New York: Grosset & Dunlop, 1940.

Articles

Ashmore, Richard D., ed. "Black and White in the 1970's", The Journal of Social Issues, 32, No. 2 (1976).

Brims, Hamilton. "The Black Family: A Proud Reappraisal." *Ebony*, March 1974, pp. 118-127.

Brunswick, Ann F. "What Generation Gap? A Comparison of Some Generational Differences among Blacks and Whites." *Social Problems*, 17 (1969-1870): 358-370.

Brunswick, Ann F., and Josephson, Eric. "Adolescent Health in Harlem," *American Journal of Public Health* 62, no. 10, pt. 2 (a separate supplement to October 1972 issue).

Bucher, K.A., Patterson, A.M., Jr.; Elston, R.C.; Jones, C.A.; and Kirkman, H., Jr. "Racial Differences in Incidence of ABO Hemolytic Disease." *American Journal of Public Health* 66 (1976): 854-858.

Cappannori, Stephen C.; Garn, Stanley M.; and Clark, Dave C. "Voodoo in the General Hospital: A Case of Regional Enteritis." *Journal of the American Medical Association* 232 (2 June, 1975): 938-940.

Carter, H. James. "Recognizing Psychiatric Symptoms in Black Americans." *Geriatrics*, November 1974, pp. 95-99.

Clark, Cedric, ed. "The White Researcher in Black Society," *The Journal of Social Issues*, 21, No. 1 (1973).

Davis, Donald. "Growing Old Black." *Employment Prospects of Aged Blacks, Chicanos and Indians*. Washington, D.C.: National Council on the Aging, 1971, pp. 27-53.

Garn, Stanley M. "Problems in the Nutritional Assessment of Black Individuals." *American Journal of Public Health* 66 (March 1976): pp. 262-267.

Grier, Marian. "Hair Care for the Black Patient." *American Journal of Nursing* 76 (November 1976): 1781.

Hess, Gertrude. "Racial Tensions: Barriers in Delivery of Nursing Care." *Journal of Nursing Administration* 5 (May-June 1972): 47-49.

"Higher Education of Minority Groups in the U.S." *Journal of Negro Education* 37 (Summer 1969): 291-303.

Houston, Susan. "Black English." *Psychology Today*, March 1973, pp. 45-48.

Jackson, J. "Aged Negroes: Their Cultural Departures from Statistical Sterotypes and Rural-urban Differences." *Gerontologist*, Summer 1970, pp. 140-145.

_____. "Kinship Relations among Negro Americans." *Journal of Social and Behavioral Sciences* 16 (1970): 5-17.

Koenig, R.; Goldner, N.S.; Kresojevich, R.; and Lockwood, G. "Ideas about Illness of Elderly Black and White in an Urban Hospital," *Aging and Human Development* 2 (1971): 217-225.

Lackler, C. "Aged Black and Poor: Three Case Studies." *Aging and Human Development* 2 (1971): 202-207.

Malina, R.M. "Skinfolds in American Negro and White Children." *Journal of American Dietetic Association* 59 (1971): 34-40.

Roach, Lora B. "Assessment: Color Changes in Dark Skin." *Nursing 77 (January 1977): 48-51.*

_____. *"Assessing Skin Changes: The Subtle and the Obvious." Nursing 74* 3 (March 1974): 64-67.

Snow, Londell F. "Folk Medical Beliefs and their Implications for Care of Patients." *Annals of Internal Medicine* 81 (July 1974): 82-96.

Staples, Robert. "Towards a Sociology of the Black Family: A Theoretical and Methodological Assessment." *Journal of Marriage and the Family* (February 1971): 119-138.

Suchman, Edward A., and Rothman, Allen. "The Utilization of Dental Services." *Milbank Memorial Fund Quarterly* 47 (1970): 56-63.

CHAPTER 11

Health and Illness in the Hispanic- American Community

Members of the Hispanic-American community have their origins in Spain, Cuba, Central and South America, Mexico, Puerto Rico, and other Spanish-speaking countries. This chapter focuses on the health and illness beliefs and practices of the Chicanos and the Puerto Ricans.

THE CHICANOS

Who are the Chicanos? In answering this question, one will surely discover who the Mexican-Americans are. What should these people be called? Depending on his socioeconomic status, his age, and the area in which he lives, a member of this large minority group will refer to himself as either a Mexican-American, Spanish American, Latin American, Latin, or Mexican.[1] The word *Chicano* is used as an "identifying umbrella that identifies all Americans of Mexican descent,"[2] hence the term is used in this book to refer to this particular cultural and ethnic group.

Chicanos, according to the 1970 census, number at least 4,532,435 people.[3] This figure is known to be an underenumeration, and in 1977 there were most likely well over 12-million Chicanos in the United States.[4] This population is rapidly increasing because of a high birth rate and both legal and illegal immigration.[5]

Background

We came to California long before the Pilgrims landed at Plymouth Rock. We settled California, and all the Southwestern part of the United States, including the States of Arizona, New Mexico, Colorado, and Texas. We built the missions and cultivated the ranches.[6]

The Chicanos have been in the United States for a long time, having moved from Mexico and later intermarrying with Indians and Spanish people in the southwestern parts of what is now the United States. Santa Fe, New Mexico, was settled in 1609. Most of the descendants of these early settlers now live in Arizona, California, Colorado, New Mexico, and Texas. A large number of Chicanos also live in Illinois, Indiana, Kansas, Michigan, Missouri, Nebraska, New York, Ohio, Utah, Washington, and Wisconsin. Most Chicanos arrived in the latter states as migrant farm workers. While located there as temporary farm workers, they found permanent jobs and stayed.[7] Contrary to the popular views that Chicanos live in rural areas, most live in urban areas.[8] According to the 1960 census, Los Angeles and Long Beach had by far the largest number of Chicanos (629,292), with San Antonio (257,090) and San Francisco-Oakland (177,239) having the second and third largest number, respectively. Today, the populations in these cities are even larger.[9] Chicanos are employed in all types of jobs; however, few have high-paying or high-status jobs in labor or management. The majority work in factories, mines, and construction; others are employed in farm work and service areas. Presently, only a small—although growing—number of the people are employed in clerical and professional areas. The number of unemployed is high (estimated to be between 25 and 35 percent), and the earnings of those employed are well below the national average. The education of Chicanos, like that of most minorities in the United States, lags behind that of most of the population. Many

Chicanos fail to complete high school. However, in the past few years, this situation has changed, and Chicano children are being encouraged to stay in school, go on to college, and enter the professions.[10]

Traditional Definitions of
Health and Illness

There are conflicting reports with reference to the traditional meaning of health. Some sources maintain that health is considered to be purely the result of "good luck" and that a person will lose his good health if his luck changes.[11] Some Chicanos describe health as a reward for good behavior; seen in this context, health is a gift from God and should not be taken for granted. People are expected to maintain their own equilibrium in the universe by performing in the proper way, eating the proper foods, and working the proper amount of time. The prevention of illness is an accepted practice that is accomplished with prayer, the wearing of religious medals or amulets, and keeping relics in the home. Herbs and spices can also be used to enhance this form of prevention, as can exemplary behavior.[12] Illness is seen as an imbalance in an individual's body or as punishment meted out for some wrongdoing. The causes of illness can be grouped into four major categories.

The Body's Imbalance

Imbalance may exist between "hot" and "cold" or "wet" and "dry." The theory of hot and cold was brought to Mexico by Spanish priests and was fused with Aztec beliefs.[13] The concept actually dates back to the early Hippocratic theory of disease and the four body "humors." The disrupted relationship between these humors is often mentioned by Chicanos as the cause of disease, and this situation will be referred to frequently in our discussion.

There are four body fluids or humors: (a) *blood*, hot and wet; (b) *yellow bile*, hot and dry; (c) *phlegm*, cold and wet; and (d) *black bile*, cold and dry. When all of these four humors are balanced, the body is healthy. When any imbalance occurs, an illness is manifested.[14] These concepts, of course, provide one way of determining the remedy for a particular illness. For example, if an illness is classified as hot, it is treated with a cold substance. A cold disease, in turn, must be treated with a hot substance. Food, beverages, animals, and people possess the characteristics of hot and cold to various degrees. Hot foods cannot be combined; they are to be eaten with cold foods. There is no general agreement as to what is a hot disease or food and what is a cold disease or food. The classification varies from person to person, and what is hot to one person may be cold to another.[15] Therefore, if a Chicano patient refuses to eat the meals offered to him in the hospital, it is wise to ask precisely what he can eat and what combinations of foods he thinks would be helpful for the existing condition. It is important to note that *hot* and *cold* do not refer to temperature, but are descriptive of a particular substance itself.

For example, after a woman delivers a baby, a hot experience, she cannot eat pork, which is considered a hot food. She must eat something cold to restore her balance. Penicillin is a hot medication; therefore, it cannot be used to treat a hot disease.[16] The major problem for the health-care provider is to *know* that the rules, so to speak, of hot and cold vary from person to person. If health-care providers understand the general nature of the hot and cold imbalance, they will be able to help the patient reveal the nature of the problem from the perspective of the patient.

Dislocation of Parts of the Body

Two examples of "dislocation" are *empacho* and *caida de la mollera.*[17]

Empacho is believed to be caused by a ball of food clinging to the wall of the stomach. Common symptoms of this illness are stomach pains and cramps. This ailment is treated by rubbing and gently pinching the spine. Prayers are recited throughout the treatment. Another, more common cause of such illness is thought to be lying about the amount of food consumed.[18]

A 20-year-old Hispanic woman experienced the acute onset of sharp abdominal pain. She complained to her friend and together they diagnosed the problem as *empacho* and treated it by massaging her stomach and waiting for the pain to dissipate. It did not and they continued folk treatment for 48 hours. When the pain did not diminish, they sought help in a nearby hospital. The diagnosis was "acute appendicitis." The young woman nearly died and was quite embarrassed when she was scolded by the physician for not seeking help sooner.

Caida de la mollera is a more serious illness. It occurs in infants and young children under 1 year who are dehydrated for one reason or another (usually because of diarrhea or severe vomiting) and whose anterios fontanelle is depressed below the contour of the skull.[19] There is much superstition and mystery surrounding this problem. Some of the poorly educated and rural people, in particular, believe that it is caused by a nurse's or physician's having touched the head of the baby. This can be understood if we take into account that (a) the fontanelle of an infant does in fact become depressed if the infant is dehydrated and (b) when physicians or nurses measure an infant's head they do touch this area. If a mother brings her baby to a physician for an examination and sees the physician touch the child's head, and if the baby gets sick thereafter with *caida de la mollera*, it might be very easy for this woman to believe it is the fault of the physician's or nurse's touch. Unfortunately, epidemics of diarrhea are common in the rural and urban areas of the Southwest, and a number of children tend to be affected. One case of severe dehydration that leads to *caida de la mollera* may create quite a stir among the people. The folk treatment of this illness has not been found to be effective. Unfortunately, babies are rarely brought to the hospital in time, and the mortality rate for this illness is high.[20]

Magic or Supernatural Causes Outside the Body

Witchcraft or possession is considered to be culturally patterned role-playing: a safe vehicle for restoring oneself. Witchcraft or possession legitimizes acting out bizarre behavior or engaging in incoherent speech.[21]

A lesser disease that is caused from outside the body is *mal ojo*. *Mal ojo* means "bad eye," and it is believed to result from excessive admiration on the part of another. General malaise, sleepiness, fatigue, and severe headache are the symptoms of this condition. The folk treatment is to find the person who has caused the illness by casting the "bad eye" and have him care for the afflicted person.[22]

Strong Emotional States

Susto is described as an illness arising from fright. It afflicts many people—males and females, rich and poor, rural dwellers and urbanites. It involves *soul loss*: the soul is able to leave the body and wander freely. This can occur while a person is dreaming, or when a person experiences a particularly traumatic event. The symptoms of the disease are as follows: (a) the person is restless while sleeping; (b) when awake, the person is listless, anorexic, and disinterested in personal appearances, which includes both clothing and personal hygiene; (c) the individual experiences a loss of strength, is depressed, and becomes introverted. The person is treated by a *curandero* (a healer to be discussed later), who coaxes the soul back into the person's body. During the healing rites the person is massaged and made to relax.[23]

Envidia

Envidia, or envy, is also considered to be a cause of illness and bad luck. Many people believe that to succeed is to fail. That is, when one's success provokes the envy of friends and neighbors, misfortune can befall him and his family. For example, a successful farmer, just as he is able to purchase extra clothing and equipment, is stricken with a fatal illness. He may well attribute the cause of this illness to the envy of his peers. There are a number of social scientists who, after much research in this area, conclude that the "low" economic and success rates of the Chicano can ostensibly be attributed to belief in *envidia*.[24]

Religious Rituals

Magicoreligious practices are quite common among the Chicano population. The more severe an illness, the more likely that these practices will be observed. There are four types of practices: (1) making promises, (2) visiting shrines, (3) offering medals and candles, and (4) offering prayers.[25] It is not unusual for the people residing near the southern border of the continental United States to return home to Mexico on religious pilgrimages. The film mentioned earlier in this book, "We Believe in Nino Fedencio," demonstrates how these pilgrimages are conducted. The lighting of candles is also a frequently observed practice. These beautiful candles made of beeswax and tallow can be purchased in many stores, particularly grocery stores and pharmacies that are located in Chicano neighborhoods. Many homes have shrines with statues and pictures of saints. The candles are lit here and prayers are recited. Some homes have altars with statues and pictures on them and are the focal point of the home.

Curanderismo

There are no specific rules for knowing who in the community uses the services of the folk healers. Not all Chicanos do, and not all Chicanos necessarily believe in such precepts. Initially, it was thought that only the poor used a folk healer or *curandero* because they were unable to get treatment from the larger, institutionalized health-care establishment. However, it now appears that the use of healers occurs widely throughout the Chicano population. Some individuals try to use healers exclusively, whereas others use them along with institutionalized care. The healers do not "advertise," but they are well known throughout the population because of informal community and kinship networks.

Curanderismo is defined as a medical system.[26] It is a coherent view with historical roots that combine Aztec, Spanish, spiritualistic, homeopathic, and scientific elements.

The *curandero* is a holistic healer; the people who seek help from him do so for social, physical, and psychological purposes. The *curandero(a)* can be either a male or female, a "specialist" or a "generalist," a full-time or part-time practitioner. Chicanos who believe in *curanderos* consider them to be religious figures.

A *curandero* may receive the "gift of healing" through three means. (1) He may be "born" to heal. In this case it is known from the moment of a *curandero's* birth that there is something unique about him and that he is destined to be a healer. (2) He may learn by apprenticeship—that is, a person is taught the ways of healing, especially the use of herbs; (3) He may receive a "calling"—through a dream, trance, or vision by which he makes contact with the supernatural via a "patron" (or "caller"), who may be a saint. The "call" comes either during adolescence or during the midlife crises. This "call" is resisted at first. Later the person resigns himself to his fate and gives in to the demands of the "calling."

Treatments

The most popular form of treatment used by folk healers involves herbs, especially when used as teas. The *curandero* knows what specific herbs to use for a problem; this information is revealed in dreams in which the "patron" gives suggestions.

Since the *curandero* has a religious orientation, much of the treatment includes elements of both the Catholic and Pentecostal rituals and artifacts: offerings of money, penance, confession, lighting candles, wooden or metal offerings in the shape of the afflicted anatomic parts (*milagros*), and laying on of hands.

Massage is used in illnesses such as *empacho* (discussed earlier), which is believed to be caused by a ball of food's clinging to the wall of the stomach. The symptoms are stomach pains and cramps and for treatment the spine is gently pinched and massaged by the healer.

Cleanings, or *limpias*, are done in two ways. The first is to pass an unbroken egg over the body of the ill person. The second method entails passing herbs tied in a bunch over the body. The back of the neck, which is considered a vulnerable spot, is given particular attention.

In contrast to the depersonalized care a Chicano expects to receive in medical institutions, his relationship with and care by the *curandero* are uniquely personal, as demonstrated in the comparative listing below. This special relationship between the Chicano and the *curandero* may well account for this folk healer's popularity. In addition to the close, personal relationship between patient and healer, there are many factors that explain the continuing belief in *curanderismo*.

1. The mind and body are inseparable.
2. The central problem of life is to maintain harmony. This includes the social as well as the physical and psychological aspects of the person.
3. There must be harmony between the hot and cold, wet and

Table 5. Comparisons: Curandero versus Physician

Curandero	Physician
1. Maintains informal, friendly, affective relationship with entire family.	1. Businesslike, formal relationship; deals only with the patient.
2. Comes to house day or night.	2. Patient must go to physician's office or clinic, and only during the day; may have to wait for hours to be seen; home visits are rarely made.
3. For diagnosis, consults with head of house, creates a mood of awe, talks to all family members, is not authoritarian, has social rapport, builds expectation of cure.	3. Rest of family is usually ignored; deals solely with the ill person, and may deal only with the sick part of the patient; authoritarian manner creates fear.
4. Is generally less expensive than physicians.	4. More expensive than *curanderos.*
5. Has ties to the "world of the sacred;" has rapport with the symbolic, spiritual, creative, or holy force.	5. Secular; pays little attention to the religious beliefs or meaning of a given illness.
6. Shares the world view of the patient—that is, speaks the same language, lives in the same neighborhood or in some similar socioeconomic conditions, may know the same people, understands the life-style of the patient.	6. Generally does not share the world view of the patient—that is, may not speak the same language, does not live in the same neighborhood, does not understand the socioeconomic conditions, does not understand the life-style of the patient.

dry. The treatment of illness should restore the body's harmony, which has been lost.

4. The patient is the passive recipient of disease when the disease is caused by an external force. This external force disrupts the natural order of the internal person, and the treatment must be designed to restore this order. The causes of disharmony are evil and witches.

5. A person is related to the spirit world; when the body and soul are separated, there can be "soul loss." This loss is sometimes caused by *susto*, a disease or illness resulting from fright, which may afflict individuals from all socioeconomic levels and lifestyles.
6. The responsibility for recovery is shared by the ill person, the family, and the *curandero*.
7. The natural world is not clearly distinguished from the supernatural world; thus the *curandero* can coerce, curse, and appease the spirits. The *curandero* places more emphasis on his connections with the sacred and his gift of healing than on personal properties. (Such personal properties might include, for example, social status, a large home, and expensive material goods.)

PUERTO RICANS

Puerto Rican migrants to the mainland are first and foremost American citizens, albeit with a different language and culture. They are neither immigrants nor aliens in the continental United States. According to the 1970 census, there are at least 1,429,396 Puerto Ricans living on the mainland. They live mostly on the East Coast, with the greatest number living in New York City and Metropolitan New Jersey. Most Puerto Ricans migrate to search for a better life or because relatives, particularly spouses and parents, have previously migrated. Life on the island of Puerto Rico is difficult because there is a high level of unemployment.[27] Puerto Ricans are not well known or understood by the majority of people in the continental United States; little is known about their cultural identity. Mainlanders tend to forget that Puerto Rico is, for the most part, a poor island and that there are many problems for the people who live there. When so many Puerto Ricans migrate to the mainland they bring many of their problems—especially those of poor health and social circumstance.[28]

Puerto Ricans, along with Cubans, comprise the most recent major immigration to these shores. They cover the spectrum of racial differences, and have practiced racial intermarriage. Many are Catholic, but some belong to various Protestant sects.

There are similarities both in the ways in which Puerto Ricans and Chicanos perceive health and illness and in the use of folk healers and remedies. There are also differences. Most studies on health and illness beliefs and healing have been done on Chicanos. It is not easy to find information about the beliefs of Puerto Ricans. Much of the information presented here was gleaned from students and patients. Both groups feel that their beliefs should be known by health-care deliverers. One student, whose mother is a healer and is teaching her daughter the art, corroborated much of the following material.

Common Folk Diseases and Their Treatment

Table 6 lists a number of folk diseases in addition to the source and type of treatment that are customarily utilized.* Many of these diseases or disharmonies have been mentioned in the section on Chicano approaches. Nonetheless, there are subtle differences in the ways that they are perceived by Chicanos and Puerto Ricans. For example, while diseases are classified as hot and cold, treatments—that is, food and medications—are categorized as hot (*caliente*), cold (*frio*), and cool (*fresco*). Cold illnesses are treated with hot remedies; hot diseases are treated with cold *or cool* remedies. Table 7 lists the major illnesses, foods, medicines, and herbs associated with the hot-cold system as it is applied among Puerto Ricans in New York.

A number of activities are carried out to maintain the proper hot-cold balance in the body. The following list was prepared by a patient:

1. *Pasmo*, a form of paralysis, is usually caused by an upset in the hot-cold balance. For example, if a woman is ironing (hot) and then steps out into the rain (cold), she may get facial or other paralyses;
2. A person who is hot cannot sit under a mango tree (cold) because he can get a kidney infection or "back problems;"
3. A baby should not be fed a formula (hot) as it may cause rashes; whole milk (cold) is acceptable;
4. A person who has been working (hot) must not go

*The data contained in Table 6 were provided by Puerto Rican students and patients who were carefully interviewed several times.

Table 6. Folk Diseases

Name	Description	Treatment	Source of Treatment
Susto	Sudden fright, causing shock	Relaxation	Relative or friend
Fatigue	Asthma-like symptoms	Oxygen; medications	"Western" health care system
Pasmo	Paralyses-like symptoms, face or limbs	Prevention; massage	Folk
Empacho	Food forms into a ball and clings to the stomach, causing pain and cramps	Strong massage over the stomach; medication; gently pinching and rubbing the spine	Folk
Mal ojo	Sudden, unexplained illness in a usually well child or person	Prevention; babies wear a special charm	Depends on the severity of the symptoms; usually home or folk
Ataque	Screaming, falling to ground, wildly moving arms and legs	None—ends spontaneously	

into the coffee fields (cold) or he can contract a
respiratory illness;

5. A hot person must not drink cold water as it could
cause colic.

There is often a considerable time lag between disregarding
these precautions and the occurrence of illness. A patient who had
injured himself while lifting heavy cartons in a factory revealed
that the "true" reason he was now experiencing prolonged back
problems was because as a child he often sat under a mango tree
when he was "hot" after running. This childhood habit had significantly damaged his back so that, as an adult, he was unable to
lift heavy objects without causing injury.

Table 8 summarizes some of the behaviors a patient may manifest with certain illnesses that are caused by the hot and cold
imbalance.

Puerto Ricans also share with others of Hispanic origin a number of beliefs in spirits and spiritualism. They believe that mental
illness is caused primarily by evil spirit and forces. People with
such disorders are preferably treated by a "spiritualist medium":[28]
the psychiatric clinic is known as the place where *locos* go. This
attitude is exemplified in the Puerto Rican approach to visions and
the like. The social and cultural environment encourages the acceptance of having visions and hearing voices. In the dominant
culture of the continental United States, when one has visions or
hears voices one is encouraged to see a psychiatrist. When a Puerto
Rican regards this experience as a problem, he may seek help
through *santeria*.[29] *Santeria* is a structured system consisting of
espiritismo, which is practiced by gypsies and mediums who claim
to have *facultades*. These special *facultades* provide them with the
"license" to practice. The positions of the practitioners form a
hierarchy: the head is the *babalow*, a male; second is the *presi-
dente*, the head medium; third are the *santeros*. Novices are the
"believers."

The *facultades* are given to the healer from protective Catholic
saints, who have African names and are known as *protecciones*.
Santeria can be practiced in storefronts, basements, homes, and
even college dormitories (as we saw in an earlier chapter). *Santeros*
dress in white robes for ceremonies and wear special beaded
bracelets as a sign of their identity.[30]

Table 7. Hot-Cold Classification among Puerto Ricans

	Frio (Cold)	Fresco (Cool)	Caliente (Hot)
Illnesses or bodily conditions	Arthritis Colds *Friaidad del estómago* * Menstrual period Pain in the joints *Pasmo*		Constipation Diarrhea Rashes Tenesmus *(pulo)* Ulcers
Medicines and herbs		Bicarbonate of soda Linden flowers *(flor de tilo)* Mannitol *(maná de manito)* Mastic bark *(almácigo)* $MgCO_3$ *(magnesia boba)* Milk of magnesia Nightshade *(yerba mora)*	Anise Aspirin Castor oil Cinnamon Cod liver oil Iron tablets Penicillin

Foods		
Avocado	Orange flower water (agua de azahar)	Rue (ruda)
Bananas	Sage	Vitamins
Coconut	Barley water	Alcoholic beverages
Lima beans	Bottled milk	Chili peppers
Sugar cane	Chicken	Chocolate
White beans	Fruits	Coffee
	Honey	Corn meal
	Raisins	Evaporated milk
	Salt cod (bacalao)	Garlic
	Watercress	Kidney beans
		Onions
		Peas
		Tobacco

From A. Harwood, "The Hot-Cold Theory of Disease: Implications for Treatment of Puerto Rican Patients," *Journal of the American Medical Association* 216 (1971): 1154-1155, copyright 1971, American Medical Association

*This describes a condition known as "cold stomach" and is caused by eating too many foods classified as "cold."

Table 8. Expectable Behavior of Patients Who Adhere to the Hot-Cold Theory

Patient's Condition	Expectable Behavior
Common cold, arthritis, joint pains	Patient will not take cold-classified foods or medications but will accept those classed as hot
Diarrhea, rash, ulcers	Patient will not take hot-classified medications and uses cool substances as therapy
Requires a diuretic as part of a treatment regimen and has been told to supplement his potassium intake by eating bananas, oranges, raisins, or dried fruit	Patient will not eat these cold-classified foods while he has a cold or other cold-classified condition (for female patients this includes the menses)
Requires penicillin or any other hot medication, particularly on an ongoing basis	Patient will stop taking hot medicine when he suffers any hot-classified symptom (e.g., diarrhea, constipation, rash)
Infant requires formula, which contains hot-classified evaporated milk	Mother will put baby on cold-classified whole milk or will, after feeding formula, "refresh" the baby's stomach with various cool substances, some of which are diuretic
Pregnant	Will avoid hot medicine and hot foods and takes cool medicine frequently
Postpartum and during menstruation	Will avoid cool foods and medicines, particularly those that are acidic

From A. Harwood, "The Hot-Cold Theory of Disease: Implications for Treatment of Puerto Rican Patients," *Journal of the American Medical Association* 216 (1971): 1154-1155, copyright 1971, American Medical Association

Puerto Ricans are able to accept much of what Anglos may judge to be idiosyncratic behavior. In fact, behavioral disturbances are seen as symptoms of illness that are to be treated, not judged.

As suggested earlier, there is a sharp distinction between "nervous" behavior and being *loco*. To be *loco* is to be bad, dangerous, evil. It also means losing all of one's social status. Puerto Ricans who seek standard American treatment for mental illness are castigated by the community; thus they understandably prefer to get help for the symptoms of mental illness from the *santero*, who accepts the symptoms and attributes the cause of the illness to spirits outside the body. Puerto Ricans have great faith in this system of care and maintain a high level of hope for recovery.[31]

The *santero* is an important person: he respects the individual and does not gossip about either the person or his problems. Anyone can "pour his heart out" with no worry of being labeled or judged. The *santero* is able to tell a person what the problem is, prescribe the proper treatment, and tell the individual what to do, how to do it, and when to do it. A study in New York found that 73 percent of the Puerto Rican patients in an out-patient mental health clinic reported having visited a *santero*.[32] Often a sick person is taken to a psychiatrist by his family to be "calmed down" and prepared for treatment by a *santero*. Families may become angry if the psychiatrist does not encourage belief in God and prayer during the time that he works with the patient.[33] Because of cultural differences and beliefs, a psychiatrist may often diagnose as illness what Puerto Ricans may define as health. Frequently, a spiritualist will treat the "mental illness" of a patient as *facultades*, which makes the patient a "special person": thus esteem is granted to the patient as a form of treatment.[34]

Entry into Health Systems

Puerto Ricans living in New York City and other parts of the northern United States experience a high rate of illness and hospitalization during their first year on the mainland,[35] as do other people of Hispanic origin. It is worthwhile considering for a moment the vast differences between living in New York and living in Puerto Rico. In Puerto Rico winter is unheard of. The winters in the north can be bitter cold, and adjustments to climate change in itself is extremely difficult. Migrant people may also be forced to live in crowded living quarters with poor sanitation.

When a Puerto Rican seeks health care, he may go to a physician or to a folk practitioner or to both. The general progression of seeking care is as follows:

1. The individual seeks advice from a daughter, mother, grandmother, or neighbor woman. These sources are consulted because the women of this culture are the primary healers and dispensers of medicine on the family level.
2. If the adivce is not sufficient, the individual may seek help from a *senoria* (a woman who is especially knowledgeable about the causes and treatment of illness).
3. If the *senoria* is unable to help the person, he goes to a more sophisticated folk practitioner, an *espiritista* or a *curandera*. If the problem is "psychiatric," a *santero* may be consulted. These names describe similar people—those who obtain their knowledge from spirits and treat illness according to the instructions of the spirits. Herbs, lotions, creams, and massage are often used.
4. If the person is still not satisfied, he may go to a physician.
5. If the results are not satisfactory, the individual may return to a folk practitioner. He may seek medical help sooner than Step 4, and/or he may go back and forth between the two systems.

Not all Puerto Ricans use the folk system. Health-care providers should remember that people who appear to have delayed seeking health care have most likely counted on curing their illness through the culturally known and well-understood folk process. Often when people disappear—or "elope" from the established health system—they may have elected to return to the folk system. Individuals who elope from the larger, institutionalized medical system may opt to visit *botanica*. There are 24 *botanicas* located in one small area of New York City. In these small *botanicas,* one can purchase herbs, potents, Florida water, ointments, and incense prescribed by the spiritualists. Some of these *botanicas* are so busy that each customer is given a number and is assisted only after his number is called.[36] A Spanish-speaking colleague and I visited a *botanica* in Boston that was similar to a pharmacy. The door was locked, but the proprietor admitted us when we revealed our identity. He explained the various remedies that were for sale. We were allowed to purchase only a few items because we did not have a spiritualist's prescription for herbs. The store also sold candles, religious statues, cards, medals, and relics.

A limited number of *santerias* place advertisements in local Spanish daily newspapers. Some of the more industrious ones distribute flyers in the New York City subways. Others maintain a low profile, and patients visit them because of their well-established reputations. I attempted to visit a *santera* in the Boston area but was unable to locate her; she had recently vacated her apartment and no one in the building would or could tell me where she had relocated.

CURRENT HEALTH PROBLEMS

There are a number of health problems that Hispanic people have in common. They experience a number of barriers when they seek health care. The most evident one is that of language. In spite of the fact that Spanish-speaking people comprise one of the largest minority groups in this country, there are very few Spanish-speaking health-care deliverers. This is especially true in communities in which there is a limited number of Spanish-speaking people; Hispanics who live in these areas experience tremendous frustration because of the language barrier. Even in large cities there are far too many occasions when a sick individual has to rely on a young child to act not only as a translator but also as interpreter. One way of sensitizing young students to the pain of this situation is to ask them to present a health problem to a person who does not speak or understand a word of English. Needless to say, this is extremely difficult; it is also embarrassing. People who try this rapidly comprehend and appreciate the feelings that are experienced by patients who are unable to speak or understand English. (After this experience two of my students decided to take a foreign-language elective: that amounts to two more concerned student nurses!) Language will continue to be a problem until

(1) there are more physicians, nurses, and social workers from the Spanish-speaking communities and (2) more of the present deliverers of health care learn to speak Spanish.

A second barrier that Hispanic people encounter is poverty: it is a crucial problem among people of Spanish origin. The diseases of the poor—for example, tuberculosis, malnutrition, and lead poisoning—all have high incidences among Spanish-speaking populations.

A final barrier to adequate health care is the time orientation of Hispanic Americans. To Hispanics, time is a relative phenomenon. Little attention is given to the *exact* time of day. The frame of reference is wider, and the issue is whether it is day or night.[37] The American health system, on the other hand, places great emphasis on promptness. Health-care providers demand that clients arrive at the exact time of the appointment—despite the fact that clients are often kept waiting. Health-system workers stress the client's promptness rather than their own. In fact, they tend to deny responsibility for the waiting periods by blaming them on the "system." Many facilities commonly schedule all appointments for 9:00 A.M. when it is clearly known and understood by the staff members that the doctor will not even arrive until 11:00 A.M. or later. The Hispanic person frequently responds to this practice by coming late for appointments or failing to come at all. They prefer to attend walk-in clinics, where the waits are shorter, and they much prefer going to the healer.

Hispanic-American Manpower

The number of Hispanic-origin Americans enrolled in health programs is low—for example, 1 percent of the 0.3 percent minority students in medical schools, 0.8 percent of the 7.5 percent minority students in dentistry, and 1 percent of the 5.9 percent minority students in optometry. In nursing programs, too, there is a limited representation of Spanish-speaking people among applicants regardless of whether the program is diploma, baccalaureate, or associate degree.

The number of practicing professionals is limited. For example, 1.1 percent of dentists, 1.6 percent of optometrists, 3.7 percent of pharmacists, and 3.7 percent of physicians (medical and osteopathic) are people of Hispanic origin. In other words, there are 11.3 dentists, 23.1 pharmacists, and 113.9 physicians of Spanish origin per 100,000 people.[38]

REFERENCES

1. Edward Simmen, ed., *Pain and Promise: The Chicano Today* (New York: Times Mirror, 1972), p. 35.
2. Ibid., p. 36.
3. Ibid., p. 46.
4. William H. McBeath et al., "Minority Health Chart Book," presented at the 102nd Annual Meeting of the American Public Health Association, New Orleans, 20-24 October, 1974, p. 1.
5. Edward Simmen and Bureau of the Census, "We Mexican Americans" (Washington, D.C.: US Government Printing Office, 19) p. 46.
6. Edward Simmen, "Anonymous, Who Am I?" in *Educating the Mexican American*, Henry Sioux Johnson and William J. Hernandez-M., eds. Valley Forge, Pa: Judson Press, 1970), p. 38.
7. Edward Simmen and Bureau of the Census, op cit.,[5] pp. 45-47.
8. Ibid., p. 47.
9. Ibid., p. 48.
10. Ibid., pp. 49-52.
11. Susan Welch, John Comer, and Michael Stlinman, "Some Social and Attitudinal Correlates of Health Care among Mexican Americans," *Journal of Health and Social Behavior* 14 (September 1973): 205.
12. Gilberto Lucero, "Health and Illness in the Chicano Community" (lecture given at Boston College School of Nursing, March, 1975).
13. Ibid.
14. Richard L. Currier, "The Hot-Cold Syndrome and Symbolic Balance in Mexican and Spanish-American Folk Medicine," *Ethnology* 5, (1966): 251-263.
15. Lyle Saunders, "Healing Ways in the Spanish Southwest" in *Patients, Physicians, and Illness*, E. Gartley Jaio, ed. (Glencoe, Ill.: Free Press, 1958), p. 193.
16. Ibid., p. 193.
17. Frank C. Nall II and Joseph Speilberg, "Social and Cultural Factors in the Responses of Mexican-Americans to Medical Treatment," *Journal of Health and Social Behavior* 8, (1967): 302.
18. Ibid., p. 302.
19. Pauline Rodriquez Dorsey and Herlinda Quinterg Jackson, "Cultural Health Traditions: The Latino/Chicano Perspective" in *Provid-*

> *ing Safe Nursing Care for Ethnic People of Color*, Marie Foster Branch and Phyllis Perry Paxton, eds. (New York: Appleton, (1976), p. 56.

20. Gilberto Lucero, op cit.[12]
21. Ibid.
22. Frank C. Nall II and Joseph Speilberg, op cit.,[17] p. 302.
23. Arthur J. Rubel, "The Epidemiology of a Folk Illness: Gusto in Hispanic America," *Ethnology* 3, no. 3 (July 1964): 270-71.
24. Gilberto Lucero, op cit.[12]
25. Frank C. Nall II and Joseph Speilberg, op cit.,[17] p. 303.
26. Renoldo J. Maduro, "Curanderismo: Latin American Folk Healing" Conference, "Ways of Healing, Ancient and Modern," San Francisco, January, 1976); Ari Kiev, *Curanderismo: Mexican-American Folk Psychiatry*, New York: Free Press, 1968; Gilberto Lucero, op cit.[12]
27. Raquel E. Cohen, "Principles of Preventive Mental Health Programs for Ethnic Minority Populations: The Acculturation of Puerto Ricans to the United States," *American Journal of Psychiatry* 128, no. 12 (June 1972): 79.
28. Ibid.
29. Emily Mumford, "Puerto Rican Perspectives on Mental Illness," *Mount Sinai Journal of Medicine* 40, no. 6 (November-December 1973): 771.
30. Ibid.
31. Ibid.
32. Ibid., p. 772.
33. Ibid., p. 773.
34. Ibid., p. 771.
35. Ibid.
36. Ibid., p. 772.
37. Gilberto Lucero, op cit.[12]
38. William McBeath et al., op cit.[4]

BIBLIOGRAPHY: HEALTH AND ILLNESS IN THE SPANISH-AMERICAN COMMUNITY

Butler, Helen. *Doctor Gringo*. New York: Rand McNally, 1967.

> This is the story of a young physician who practices modern medicine in a remote village in Mexico. It aptly describes the differences between the cultural beliefs of the people and standard American medicine.

Kiev, Ari. *Curanderismo: Mexican-American Folk Psychiatry*. New York: Free Press, 1968.

> Kiev presents an in-depth study of Mexican-American folk

psychiatry in San Antonio, Texas. In this study, the folk healers' sensitivity to the nuances and subtleties of psychopathology among members of his group are examined.

Lewis, Oscar. *A Death in the Sanchez Family.* New York: Random House, 1966.

_____. *The Children of Sanchez: Autobiography of a Mexican Family.* New York: Random House, 1961.

_____. Five Families: *Mexican Case Studies in the Culture of Poverty.* New York: New American Library, 1959.

_____. *La Vida: A Puerto Rican Family in the Culture of Poverty.* New York: Random House, 1966.

The works of Oscar Lewis, each in its own way, portray a "slice of life" of the people he observed. The books are very relevant and helpful in the context of cultural diversity in health care.

Padilla, Elena. *Up from Puerto Rico.* New York: Columbia University Press, 1958.

This book describes the Puerto Rican migration to New York City and explores the issues inherent in a large migration of people.

Rand, Christopher. *The Puerto Ricans.* New York: Oxford University Press, 1958.

The contrasts between living in New York City and living in Puerto Rico are explored in this book.

Rogler, Lloyd H. *Migrant in the City.* New York: Basic Books, 1972.

Rogler relates the story of a Puerto Rican action group and how it involved people who came from Puerto Rican slums to New York.

Simmen, Edward, editor. *Pain and Promise: The Chicano Today.* New York: New American Library, 1972.

Vivid, sensitive accounts of the reawakening of a proud and oppressed people are presented. The book consists of numerous essays—written mainly by Chicanos—that explore the identity and life problems of the people.

Steiner, Stan. *La Raza: The Mexican Americans.* New York: Harper, 1969.

This book consists of essays, short stories, and poetry illustrating the life and beliefs of the Chicano people.

Thomas, Piri. *Down These Mean Streets.* New York: Signet, 1958.

_____. *Savior, Savior, Hold my Hand.* Garden City, N.Y.: Doubleday, 1972.

Both these books depict life in the streets of Harlem as experienced by the writer.

FURTHER SUGGESTED READINGS

Books

Chenault, Lawrence R. *The Puerto Rican Migrant in New York City.* New York: Columbia University Press, 1938.

Clark, Margaret. *Health in the Mexican-American Culture: A Community Study.* Berkeley and Los Angeles: University of California Press, 1959.

Coles, Robert. *Uprooted Children: The Early Life of Migrant Farm Workers.* Pittsburgh: University of Pittsburgh Press, 1970.

Farge, Emile J. *La Vida Chicana: Health Care Attitudes and Behaviors of Houston Chicanos.* San Fransisco: Robert D. Reed, 1975.

Harwood, Alan. *Rx: Spiritist as Needed—A Study of a Puerto Rican Community Mental Health Resource.* New York: Wiley, 1977.

Moquin, Wayne. *A Documentary History of the Mexican Americans.* New York: Praeger, 1972.

Saunders, Lyle. *Cultural Differences and Medical Care: The Case of the Spanish-Speaking People of the Southwest.* New York: Russell Sage Foundation, 1954.

Senior, Clarence. *The Puerto Ricans: Strangers—Then Neighbors.* Chicago: Quadrangle Books, 1961.

Sexton, Patricia Cayo. *Spanish Harlem.* New York: Harper, 1965.

Articles

Abril, I. "Mexican American Folk Beliefs That Affect Health Care." *Arizona Nurse* 28 (May-June 1975): 14-20.

Aguirre, Lydia R. "The Meaning of the Chicano Movement." In *We Are Chicanos.* Edited by P.D. Orrego. New York: Washington Square, 1973.

Baca, Josephine. "Some Health Beliefs of the Spanish-speaking." *American Journal of Nursing* (October 1969): 2172-2176.

Bace, J.E. "Some Health Beliefs of the Spanish-speaking." *American Journal of Nursing* (October 1972): 1852-1854.

Cohen, Raquel. "Principles of Preventive Mental Health Programs for Ethnic Minority Populations: The Acculturation of Puerto Ricans to the United States." *American Journal of Psychiatry* 128 (June 1972): 79-83.

Currier, Richard. "The Hot-Cold Syndrome and Symbolic Balance in Mexican and Spanish-American Folk Medicine." Ethonology 5 (1966): 251-253.

Fabrega, Horacio, Jr. "On the Specificity of Folk Illness." *Southwestern Journal of Anthropology* 29 (1970): 305-314.

Fernandez-Marina, Ramon; Maldonado-Sierra, Eduardo; and Trent, Richard D. "Three Basic Themes in Mexican and Puerto Rican Family Values." *Journal of Social Psychology* 48 (1958): 167-181.

Garrison, Vivian. "Doctor, *Espiritista,* or Psychiatrist? Health-Seeking Behavior in a Puerto Rican Neighborhood in New York City." *Medical Anthropology* 1 (1977): 65-180.

_____. "The 'Puerto Rican Syndrome' in Psychiatry and *Espiritismo.*" In *Case Studies in Spirit Possession.* Edited by Vincent Crapanzano and Vivian Garrison. New York: Wiley, 1977.

Harwood, Alan, "The Hot-Cold Theory of Disease." *Journal of the American Medical Association* 216 (17 May 1971): 1153-1158.

Hoppe, Sue Keir, and Heller, Peter L. "Alienation, Familism, and the Utilization of Health Services by Mexican Americans." *Journal of Health and Social Behavior* 16 (September 1975): 304-314.

Koss, Joan, "Therapeutic Aspects of Puerto Rican Cult Practices." *Psychiatry* 38 (1975): 160-171.

_____. "Social Process, Healing and Self-Defeat among Puerto Rican Spiritists." *American Ethnologist* 4 (1977): 453-469.

Lauria, Anthony, Jr. " 'Respeto,' 'Rela Jo' and Interpersonal Relations in Puerto Rico." *Anthropological Quarterly* 5 (April 1964): 53-67.

Lawrence, T.F.L.; Bozzetti, L.; and Kane, T.J. "Curanderas, A Unique Role for Mexican Women." *Psychiatric Annals* 2 (February 1976): 65-73.

Martinez, C. and Martin, Harry. "Folk Diseases among Urban Mexican Americans." *Journal of the American Medical Association* 196 (11 April 1966): 147-150.

Mumford, Emily. "Puerto Rican Perspectives on Mental Health." *Mount Sinai Journal of Medicine* 40 (November-December 1973): 768-779.

Nall, Frank C., II, and Speilberg, Joseph. "Social and Cultural Factors in the Responses of Mexican-Americans to Medical Treatment" *Journal of Health and Social Behavior* 8 (1967): 299-308.

Olesen, Virginia, and Hayes-Bautista, David E. "A Myth Destroyed: Chicanos Care About Health." *New Physician* (February 1973): 81-85.

Phillipos, M.J. "Successful and Unsuccessful Approaches to Mental Health Services for an Urban Hispano American Population." *American Journal of Public Health* 61 (April 1971): 820-830.

Rogler, Lloyd H., and Hollingshead, August B. "The Puerto Rican Spiritualist as a Psychiatrist." *American Journal of Sociology* 5 (July 1961): 17-21.

Rubel, Arthur J. "Concepts of Disease in Mexican-American Culture." *American Anthropologist* 62 (October 1960): 795-814.

_____. "The Epidemiology of a Folk Illness: Susto in Hispanic America." *Ethnology* 6 (July 1964): 268-282.

Russell, George, Associate Ed. "It's your Turn in the Sun." *Time* 112, No. 16 (Oct. 16, 1978): 48-61.

Saunders, Lyle. "Healing Ways in the Spanish Southwest." In *Patients, Physicians, and Illness.* Edited by E. Gartley Jaco. Glencoe, Ill.: Free Press, 1958.

Staton, Ross D. "A Comparison of Mexican and Mexican-American Families."
    Family Coordinator 21 (July 1972): 325-329.
Weaver, Jerry L. "Mexican American Health Care Behavior: A Critical Review
    of the Literature." *Social Science Quarterly* 54 (June 1973):
    85-102.
Weaver, Thomas. "Use of Hypothetical Situations in a Study of Spanish
    American Illness Referral Systems." *Human Organization,*
    Summer 1970, pp. 140-154.
Welch, Susan; Comer, John; and Steinman, Michael. "Some Social and
    Attitudinal Correlates of Health Care among Mexican Ameri-
    cans." *Journal of Health and Social Behavior* 14 (September
    1975): 205-213.

CHAPTER 12

Health and Illness in the Native-American Community

To be an Indian in modern American society is in a very real sense to be unreal and antihistorical.

—Vine Deloria

To realize the plight of today's American Indian, it is necessary to take a journey back in time to the years when whites settled in this land. Before the arrival of Europeans, this country had no name but was owned and inhabited by groups of people who called themselves nations. The people were strong both in their knowledge of the land and in their might as warriors. The Vikings reached the shores of this country about 1010 A.D. They were unable to settle on the land and left after a decade of frustration. Much later, another group of settlers were repulsed and have since been termed the "Lost Colonies." However, more and more people came to these shores, and in rapid order the land was taken over by Europeans. As the settlers expanded westward, they signed "treaties of peace" or "treaties of land cession" with the Indians. These treaties were similar to those struck between nations, although in this case it was "big" nation versus "small" nation. One reason for treaties was to legitimize the takeover of the land that the Europeans had "discovered." Once the land was "discovered." it was divided among the Europeans, who set out to create a "legal" claim to it. The Indians signed the resultant treaties, ceding small amounts of their land to the settlers and keeping the rest for themselves. As time passed, the number of whites rapidly grew and the number of Indians diminished because of wars and disease. As these events occurred, the treaties began to lose their meaning; the Europeans came to consider them as nothing but a joke. They decided that these "natives" had no real claim to the land and shifted them around like cargo from one reservation to another. Although the Indians tried to seek just settlements through court litigation, they failed to win back the land that had been taken from them through misrepresentation. For example, by 1831 the Cherokees were fighting in the court system to keep their nation in Georgia. However, they lost, and, like other Indian nations since the time of the early European settlers, were forced to move westward. During this forced westward movement many Indians died and all suffered. Today many tribes are seeking to reclaim their land through the courts, but as of 1978 the outcome is still uncertain.[1]

As the Indians migrated westward, they carried with them the fragments of their culture. Their lives were disrupted, their land was lost, and many of their leaders and teachers had perished. Yet much of their history and culture somehow remain. Today, more and more Indians are seeking to know their history. The story of the colonization and settlement of the United States is being retold with a different emphasis.

There are approximately 200 Indian tribes in the United States. Native Americans live predominantly in 26 states, with most residing in the western part of the country as a result of the forced westward migration. Although many Indians remain on reservations and in rural areas, just as many of them live in cities, especially those on the West Coast. Oklahoma, Arizona, California, New Mexico, and Alaska have the largest numbers of Native Americans.[2]

TRADITIONAL DEFINITIONS OF HEALTH AND ILLNESS

The material in this section must be regarded by the reader as being only general. This perspective is suggested because each nation or tribe had its own history and belief system regarding health and illness and the traditional treatment of illness. Yet some general beliefs and practices underlie the more specific tribal ones and every effort has been made to present them. Certain specifics are noted from time to time, either in the text or in footnotes. The data—collected through a review of the literature and from interviews granted by members of the groups known by me—come from the Navaho nation, the Hopis, the Cherokees, the Shoshones, and New England Indians with whom I have worked closely.

The traditional Native-American belief about health is that it reflects living in total harmony with nature and having the ability to survive under exceedingly difficult circumstances.[3] Humankind has an intimate relationship with nature.[4] * The earth is considered to be a living organism—the body of a higher individual, with a will and a desire to be well. The earth is periodically healthy and less healthy, just as human beings are. According to the Native-American belief system, a person should treat his body with respect, just as he should treat the earth with respect. When he harms the earth he harms himself and, conversely, when he harms himself he harms the earth.[5] The earth gives food, shelter, and medicine to humankind and, for this reason, all things of the earth belong to human beings and nature. "The land belongs to life, life belongs to the land, and the land belongs to itself." In order to maintain himself, the Indian must maintain his relationship with nature. "Mother Earth" is the friend of the Indian, and the land belongs to the Indian.[6]

According to Indian belief, as explained by Rolling Thunder, the human body is divided into two halves: these halves are seen as

---

*This philosophy was also described in a lecture at Boston College School of Nursing by Will Basque, a Mic Mac Indian and former president of the Boston Indian Council, in April 1975.

plus and minus (yet another version of the concept that every whole is made of two opposite halves). There are also—in every whole—two energy poles: positive and negative. The energy of the body can be controlled by spiritual means. It is further believed that every being has a purpose and an identity. Every being has the power to control his own self, and from this force and the belief in its potency the spiritual power of a person is kindled.[7]

Many Native Americans with traditional orientations believe that there is a reason for every sickness or pain. They believe that it is a price that is being paid, either for something that happened in the past or for something that will happen in the future. In spite of this conviction, a sick person must still be cared for. Everything is seen as being the result of something else, and this cause-and-effect relationship creates an eternal chain. Native Americans do not subscribe to the germ theory of modern medicine. Illness is something that must *be*. Even the person who is experiencing the illness may not realize the reason for its occurrence,[8] but it may, in fact, be the best possible price to pay for the past or future event(s).

The Hopi Indians associate illness with evil spirits. The evil spirit responsible for the illness is identified by the medicine man, and the remedy for the malady resides in the treatment of the evil spirit.[9]

According to legend, the Navaho people originally emerged from the depths of the earth—fully formed as human beings. Before the beginning of time, they existed with holy people, supernatural beings with supernatural powers, in a series of 12 underworlds. The creation of all elements took place in these underworlds, and there all things were made to interact in constant harmony. A number of ceremonies and rituals were created at this time for "maintaining, renewing, and mending this state of harmony."[10]

When the Navaho people emerged from the underworlds, one female was missing. She was subsequently found by a search party in the same hole from which they had initially emerged. She told the people that she had chosen to remain there and wait for their return. She became known as death, sickness, and witchcraft. Because her hair was unraveled and her body was covered with dry red ochre, the Navahos today continue to unravel the hair of their dead and to cover their bodies with red ochre. Members of the

Navaho nation believe that "witchcraft exists and that certain humans, known as witches, are able to interact with the evil spirits and that these people can bring sickness and other unhappiness to the people who annoy them."[11]

Traditionally, illness, disharmony, and sadness are seen by the Navahos as the result of one or more combinations of the following actions: "(1) displeasing the holy people; (2) annoying the elements; (3) disturbing animal and plant life; (4) neglecting the celestial bodies; (5) misuse of a sacred Indian ceremony; or (6) tampering with witches and witchcraft."[12] If disharmony exists, disease can occur. The Navahos distinguish between two types of disease: (1) contagious diseases such as measles, smallpox, diphtheria, syphilis, and gonorrhea and (2) more generalized illnesses such as "body fever" or "bodyache." The notion of illness's being caused by a microbe or other physiologic agent is alien to the Navahos. The cause of disease, of injury to a person or to his property, or of continued misfortune of any kind must be traced back to an action that should not have been performed. Examples of such infractions are breaking a taboo or contacting a ghost or witch. To the Navahos the treatment of an illness, therefore, must be concerned with the external causative factor(s) and not with the illness or injury itself.[13]

TRADITIONAL METHODS OF HEALING

Traditional Healers

The traditional healer of the Native American is the medicine man, and the Indians, by and large, have maintained their faith in him over the ages. He is a person wise in the ways of the land and of nature. He knows well the interrelationships of human beings, the earth, and the universe. He knows the ways of the plants and animals, the sun, the moon, and the stars. The medicine man takes his time to determine first the cause of the illness and then the proper treatment. In order to determine the cause and treatment of an illness, he performs special ceremonies that may take up to several days.

As a specific example, Boyd describes the medicine man, spiritual leader, philosopher, and acknowledged spokesman of the Cherokee and Shoshone tribes, Rolling Thunder, as being able to determine the cause of illness when the ill person does not himself know it. The "diagnostic" phase of the treatment may often take as long as three days. There are numerous causes of physical illness and a great number of reasons—good and/or bad—for having become ill. These causes are of a spiritual nature. When a modern physician sees a sick person, he recognizes and diagnoses only the physical illness. The medicine man, on the other hand, looks for the spiritual cause of the problem. To the Native American, "every physical thing in nature has a spiritual nature because the whole is viewed as being essentially spiritual in nature."[14] The agents of nature, herbs, are seen as spiritual helpers and the characteristics of plants must be known and understood.[14] Rolling Thunder states that "we are born with a purpose in life and we have to fulfill that purpose."[15] The purpose of the medicine man is to cure; and his power is not dying out.[15]

The medicine man of the Hopi Indians uses meditation in determining the cause of an illness, and sometimes he may even use a crystal ball as his focal point for meditation. At other times the Hopi medicine man chews on the root of jimsonweed. This powerful herb sends him into a trance as he meditates. The Hopis claim that this herb gives the medicine man a vision of the evil that caused a sickness. Once the medicine man concludes his meditation, he is able to prescribe the proper herbal treatment. For example, one illness, fever, is cured by a plant that smells like lightning; the Hopi phrase for fever is "lightning sickness."[16]

As previously stated, the Navaho Indians consider disease to result from breaking a taboo or the attack of a witch. The exact cause is diagnosed by divination, as is the ritual of treatment. There are three types of divination: motion in the hand (the most common form and often practiced by women); stargazing; and listening. The function of the diagnostician is first to determine the cause of the illness and than to recommend the treatment— that is, the type of chant that will be effective and the medicine man who can best do it. A medicine man may be called upon to treat obvious symptoms, whereas the diagnostician is called upon to ascertain the cause of the illness. (A person is considered wise if the diagnostician is called first.) Often, the same medicine man can practice both divination (diagnosis) and the sing (treat-

ment). When any form of divination is used in making the diagnosis, the diagnostician meets with the family and discusses the
patient's condition and determines the fee.

The practice of motion in the hand includes the following
rituals. Pollen and/or sand are sprinkled around the sick person,
during which time the diagnostician sits with closed eyes and with
his face turned from the patient. His hand begins to move during
the song. While the hand is moving, the diagnostician thinks of
various diseases and various causes. When the arm begins to move
in a certain way, the diagnostician knows that he has discovered
the right disease and its cause. He is then able to prescribe the
proper treatment.[17] The ceremony of motion in the hand may
also incorporate the use of dry paintings. (These paintings are a
well-known form of art.) Four colors are used—white, blue, yellow,
and black—and each color has a symbolic meaning. Chanting is
performed as the painting is produced, and the shape of the
painting determines the cause and treatment of the illness. The
chants may continue for an extended period of time,[18] depending
on the family's ability to pay and the capabilities of the singer.
The process of motion in the hand can be neither inherited nor
learned: it comes to a person suddenly, as a gift. It is said that if
an individual is able to diagnose his own illness, he is able to
practice motion in the hand.[19]

Unlike motion in the hand, stargazing can and must be learned.
Sand paintings are often, but not always, made during stargazing.
If they are not made it is either because the sick person cannot
afford to have one done or because there is not enough time to
make one. The stargazer prays the star prayer to the star spirit,
asking it to show him the cause of the illness. During stargazing,
singing begins and the star throws a ray of light that determines
the cause of the patient's illness. If the ray of light is white or
yellow the patient will recover; if it is red, the illness is serious.
If a white light falls on the patient's home, he will recover; if the
home is dark, the patient will die.[20]

Listening, the third type of divination, is somewhat similar to
stargazing, except that something is heard rather than seen. In this
instance, the cause of the illness is determined by the sound that
is heard. If someone is heard to be crying, the patient will die.[21]

The traditional Navahos continue to use the medicine man,
whom they call the singer, when an illness occurs. They use his

service because, in many instances, the treatment that they receive from him is better than the treatment they receive from the establishment. Some of the treatment modalities utilized by the singer include massage and heat treatment, the sweatbath, and use of the yucca root—approaches similar to those common in physiotherapy.[22]

The main effects of the singer are psychological. During the chant, the patient feels that he is being cared for in a deeply personal way, that he is the center of the singer's attention, and that his problem is the reason for the singer's presence. When the singer tells the patient that he will recover and the reason for his illness, he has faith in what he hears. The singer is regarded as a distinguished authority and as a person of eminence with the gift of learning from the holy people. He is considered to be more than a mere mortal. The ceremony—surrounded by such high levels of prestige, mysticism, and power—takes the sick person into its circle; he ultimately becomes one with the holy people by participating in the sing that is held in his behalf. He once again comes into harmony with the universe and subsequently becomes free of all ills and evil.[22]

The religion of the Navahos is one of *good hope* when they are sick or suffer other misfortunes. Their system of beliefs and practices helps them through the crises of life and death. The stories that are told during religious ceremonies give the people a glimpse of a world that has gone by, which promotes a feeling of security because they see that they are links in the unbroken chain of countless generations.[23]

Many Navahos believe in witchcraft, and when it is considered to be the cause of an illness special ceremonies are employed to rid the individual of the evil caused by the witches. There are numerous methods employed to manipulate the supernatural. Although many of these activities may meet with strong social disapproval, Navahos recognize the usefulness of blaming witches for illness and misfortune. Countless tales abound concerning witchcraft and how the witches work. Not all Navahos believe in witchcraft, but for those who do it provides a mechanism for laying blame for the overwhelming hardships and anxieties of life.

Such events as going into a trance can be ascribed to the work of witches. The way to cure a "witched" person is through the use of complicated prayer ceremonies that are attended by numerous friends and relatives, who lend help and express sympathy. The victim of a witch is in no way responsible for being sick and is therefore free of any punitive action by the community if his illness causes him to behave in strange ways.[24] On the other hand, if an incurably "witched" individual is affected so that alterations in his established role severely disrupt the community, he may be abandoned.

Traditional Remedies

In the past American Indians practiced an act of purification in order to maintain their harmony with nature and to cleanse the body and spirit. This was done by total immersion in water in addition to the use of sweat lodges, herb medicines, and special rituals. Today the practice is confined to total immersion of the body. Purification is seen as the first step in the control of consciousness, a ritual that awakens the body and the senses and prepares a person for meditation. It is viewed by the participants as a new beginning.[25]

As mentioned earlier, the basis of therapy lies in nature: hence the use of herbal remedies. There are specific rituals to be followed when herbs are gathered. Each plant is picked to be dried for later use. No plant is picked unless it is the proper one, and only enough plants are picked to meet the needs of the gatherers. Timing is crucial and the procedures are meticulously followed. So deep is their belief in the harmony of human beings and nature that the herb gatherers exercise great care not to disturb any of the other plants and animals in the environment.[26]

One plant of interest is the common dandelion. This plant, which contains a milky juice in its stem, is said to increase the flow of milk from the breasts of nursing mothers. Another plant, the thistle, is said to contain a substance that will relieve the prickling sensation in the throats of people who live in the desert. The medicine used to hasten the birth of a baby is called a "weasel medicine" because the weasel is clever at digging through and out of difficult territory.[27]

The following is a list of common ailments and herbal treatments used by the Hopi Indians.[28]

1. Cuts and wounds are treated with globe mallow. The root of this plant is chewed to help mend broken bones.
2. To keep air from cuts, piñon gum is applied to the wound. It is also used in an amulet to protect a person from witchcraft.
3. Cliff rose is used to wash wounds.
4. Boils are brought to a head with the use of sand sagebrush.
5. Spider bites are treated with sunflower. The person bathes in water in which the flowers have been soaked.
6. Snakebites are treated with the bladder pod. The bitter root of this plant is chewed and then placed on the bite.
7. Lichens are used to treat the gums. They are ground to a powder and then rubbed on the affected areas.
8. Fleabane is used to treat headaches. The entire herb is either bound to the head or drunk as a tea.
9. Digestive disorders are treated with blue gillia. The leaves are boiled in water and drunk to relieve indigestion.
10. The stem of the yucca plant is used as a laxative. The purple flower of the thistle is used to expel worms.
11. Blanket flower is the diuretic used to provide relief from painful urination.
12. A tea is made from painted cup and drunk to relieve the pain of menstruation. Winter fat provides a tea from the leaves and roots and is drunk if the uterus fails to contract properly during labor.

Current Health-Care Problems

Today, Native Americans are faced with a tremendous number of health-related problems. Many of the old ways of diagnosing and treating illness have not survived the migration and changing ways of the people. Because these skills have often been lost and because modern health-care facilities are not always available, the people are frequently in limbo when it comes to obtaining adequate health care. At least one-third of the Native-American population exists in a state of abject poverty. With this destitution come poor living conditions and its attendant problems, as well as diseases of the poor—including malnutrition, tuberculosis, and high maternal and infant death rates. Poverty and isolated living situations serve as further barriers that keep Native Americans from using limited health-care facilities even when they are available. Many of the illnesses that are familiar among white patients may manifest differently in Indian patients. For example, an Indian may have a high blood sugar level, yet be asymptomatic for diabetes mellitus; still, the death rate for diabetes is high among pregnant Indian women.[29]

Native Americans have the highest infant mortality rate in the United States even though their birth rate is almost twice the rate of the general population. The *neonatal* death rate has been substantially reduced; however, the *postneonatal* rate is 2.3 times that for infants of all other races. This high rate is accounted for by the marked incidence of diarrhea in young babies and the harsh environment in which they must live.

The leading causes of death in the Indian population are accidents, suicide, diabetes, alcoholism, and homicide.[30] In fact, the incidence of suicide in young Indian males is of epidemic proportions; 72 percent of all teenage suicide victims under the age of 15 are Indians.[31]

More than 50 percent of Native Americans live in urban areas. In Seattle there are 15,000 Indians. This is not a particularly dense population, but there are high rates of diphtheria; tuberculosis; otitis media, with subsequent hearing defects; alcohol abuse; inadequate immunization; iron-deficiency anemia; childhood developmental lags; mental-health problems, including depression, anxiety, and coping difficulties; and caries and other dental problems. As in all disorganized family units there are family problems related to marital difficulties and financial strain, which are usually brought about by unemployment and the lack of education or knowledge of special skills. The tension is often further compounded by alcoholism.[32]

In Boston, there are between 3,500 and 4,000 Indians. They

experience the same problems as Native Americans in other cities. Yet there is an additional problem. Few non-Indian residents are even aware that there is a Native-American community in the city or that it is in desperate need of adequate health and social services.[33]

Some historical differences in health care relate to geographical locations. For example, Indians living in the eastern part of this country and in most urban areas are *not* covered by the services of the Indian Health Service. Native Americans living on reservations in the Western portion of this country are eligible for such services. In 1923 tribal government—under the control of the Bureau of Indian Affairs—was begun by the Navahos. Treaties were established by the Navahos with the U.S. government, but in the areas of health and education, these treaties were not honored by the United States. Health services on the reservations were inadequate; consequently the people were sent to outside institutions for the treatment of illnesses such as tuberculosis and mental-health problems. As recently as 1930 the vast Navaho lands had only seven hospitals with 25 beds each. Not until 1955 were Indians finally offered concentrated services with "modern" physicians. Only since 1965 have more comprehensive services been available to the Navahos.[34]

The Indian Health Service provides in-patient facilities and out-patient clinics. There are, for example well-baby clinics, prenatal clinics, and diabetes clinics, in addition to public-health nursing services. There are community health representatives who are tribal members and who serve in the community to identify health problems, encourage people to use existing medical facilities, and take people to the clinic when the need arises.

The Indian Health Service also makes provisions for health education. Paraprofessionals and professionals in the community work in the community to educate the people, both formally and informally, in the area of current modern health practices. A section of the Indian Health Service is concerned with alcohol abuse and mental-health problems. These mental-health workers act as liaisons between the Indians and half-way houses, counselors, drug-preventive programs, and other agencies set up specifically to deal with the emotional problems of anxiety and depression. The Indian Health Service also maintains an otitis media program in view of the statistically established high incidence of this disorder among Native Americans. Young children are screened in an effort to institute early treatment so that deafness can be prevented.[35]

The ineligibility of Native Americans living on the East Coast to secure such services* has caused numerous difficulties for the needy. The providers of health care generally seem to think that Indians should receive health services from the Indian Health Service and try to send them there. However, as there simply is no Indian Health Service on the East Coast, these Native Americans tend to be shifted around among the various health-care resources that are available.

Another factor that many providers of health care and social services are not aware of is that many of the Indians on the East Coast have dual citizenship as a result of the Jay Treaty of 1794, which allows for international citizenship between the United States and Canada. This raises questions whether Indians can freely cross the border between the United States and Canada, and if those who live in the United States are eligible for welfare or medicaid if they need it.[36]

There is yet another important factor that inhibits the Indian use of white-dominated health services. The problem is a deep, cultural one: Indians suffer dis-ease when they come into contact with the white health-care provider. † Native Americans believe this because for too many years they have been the victim of haphazard care and disrespectful treatment. And all too often there is conflict between what the Native Americans perceive their illness to be and what the physician may diagnose. Native Americans, like most people, do not enjoy long waits in clinics; the separation from their families; the unfamiliar, regimental environment of the hospital; or the unfamiliar behavior of the nurses and physicians, who often display dismeaning and demanding attitudes. The response to this treatment varies. Sometimes it is silence; other times it is to leave

---

*The situation stems from the Indian Renewal Act of 1840 and the Dawes Act of 1887, legislation that disbanded tribes east of the Mississippi and established reservations west of the Mississippi.

†Dr. Red Horse[37] explains the phenomenon of "Indian paranoia" that emerges in a predictable behavior: "It is *not* a sickness but an 'interactive reality' that Native Americans suffer whenever visits to non-Indian clinics are imminent. *Fear* is a variable and often when the fear is too great, help is not sought. For example, if a Native American child has a toothache, the parents may not take the child to the dentist because they fear the dentist's demeaning attitude."

and not return. Many Native Americans request that, if the ailment is not an emergency, they be allowed to see the medicine man first and then receive treatment from the physician. Often when a sick person is afraid of receiving the care of a physician, the medicine man encourages him to go to the hospital.[38]

Specific Issues of Communication with Native Americans

There are several factors that health-care providers must be aware of when they communicate with the Native American. One of them is recognition of the importance of nonverbal communication. Often the Native American will be observing the provider and say very little; he may expect the provider to deduce the problem through instinct rather than by the extensive use of questions during history-taking. In part, this derives from the belief that direct quoting is intrusive upon individual privacy. When examining a Native American with an obvious cough, the provider might be well advised to use a declarative statement—e.g., "You have a cough that keeps you awake at night"—and then allow time for the client to respond to the statement.

It is Indian practice to converse in a very low tone of voice. It is expected that the listener will pay attention, and listen carefully in order to hear what is being said. It is considered impolite to say, "Huh?" "I beg your pardon," or to give any indication that the communication was not heard. Therefore, an effort should be made to speak with clients in a quiet setting where they will be heard more easily.

Note-taking is also taboo. Indian history has been passed through generations by means of verbal story telling. Native Americans are sensitive about note-taking while they are speaking. When one is taking a history or interviewing, it may be preferable to use memory skills rather than to record notes. This more conversational approach may encourage greater openness between the client and the provider.

Another factor to be acknowledged is the differing perceptions of time between the Native-American client and the provider. Life on the reservation is not governed by the clock, but by the dictates of need. When an Indian moves from the reservation to an urban area, he is often stressed by problems resulting from this cultural conflict concerning time. This is often encountered in delivery of health care when some Native Americans may be late for specific appointments. One viable alternative is the use of walk-in clinics.

Native-American Manpower

Throughout the nation *there are fewer than 50 Native-American doctors, fewer than 5 Native-American dentists, and only an estimated 400 Native-American nurses.*[39]

These shocking figures speak so eloquently as to preclude commentary.

REFERENCES

1. Alan Jon Fortney, "Has White Man's Lease Expired?" *New England* (*Boston Sunday Globe*), 23 January 1977, pp. 8-30; Dee Brown, *Bury My Heart at Wounded Knee* (New York: Holt, 1970); Vine Deloria, Jr., *Custer Died for Your Sins* (New York: Macmillan, 1969); and *Behind the Trail of Broken Treaties* (New York: Delacorte, 1974).
2. Martha H. Primeaux, "American Indian Health Care Practices: A Cross-Cultural Perspective," *Nursing Clinics of North America* 12, no. 1 (March 1977): 57.
3. Ibid., p. 60.
4. Doug Boyd, *Rolling Thunder* (New York: Random House, 1974), p. 96.
5. Ibid., p. 51.
6. Ibid., p. 96.
7. Ibid., p. 199.
8. Ibid., p. 123.
9. Sybil Leek, *Herbs: Medicine and Mysticism* (Chicago: Henry Regnery, 1975), p. 16.
10. Harry Bilagody, "An American Indian Looks at Health Care," in *The Ninth Annual Training Institute for Psychiatrist-Teachers of Practicing Physicians*, ed. Raymond Feldman and Dorothy Buch (Boulder: WICHE, NO. 3A30, 1969), p. 21.
11. Ibid., p. 22.
12. Ibid., p. 21.
13. Clyde Kluckhohn and Dorothea Leighton, *The Navaho*, rev. ed. (Garden City, New York: Doubleday, 1962), pp. 192-193.
14. Doug Boyd, op cit.,[4] p. 124.
15. Ibid., p. 263.

16. Sybil Leek, op cit.,[9] p. 16.
17. Leland C. Wyman, "Navaho Diagnosticians," in *Medical Care*, ed. W. Richard Scott and Edmund H. Volkhart (New York: Wiley, 1966), pp. 8-14.
18. Clyde Kluckhohn and Dorothea Leighton, op cit.,[13] pp. 209-218.
19. Leland Wyman, op cit.,[17] p. 14.
20. Ibid., p. 15.
21. Ibid., p. 16.
22. Clyde Kluckhohn and Dorothea Leighton, op cit.,[13] p. 230.
22. Ibid., p. 232.
23. Ibid., p. 233.
24. Ibid., p. 244.
25. Doug Boyd, op cit.,[4] pp. 97-100.
26. Ibid., pp. 101-136.
27. Sybil Leek, op cit.,[9] p. 17.
28. Ibid., pp. 17-26.
29. Ernestine Huffman White, "Call of the Minority Patients," *Nursing Clinics of North America* 12, no. 1 (March 1977).
30. Martha Primeaux, op cit.,[2] pp. 58-59.
31. Ernestine Huffman White, op cit.,[29] p. 36.
32. "What are the Problems of Urban Native Americans?" (flyer distributed by the Seattle Indian Health Board, 1131 14th Avenue South, Seattle, Wash., 98122, 1974).
33. John Ginnish, Lecture given at Boston College School of Nursing, April 9, 1975, "The Health Needs of the Boston Indian."
34. Harry Bilagody, op cit.,[10] pp. 22-23.
35. John Ginnish, op cit.[33]
36. Ibid.
37. John Red Horse, "Urban Native American Health Care" (Minneapolis-St. Paul: Unpublished paper, 1976), p. 3.
38. Harry Bilagody, op cit.,[10] p. 22; John Ginnish, op cit. [33]
39. "What are the Problems?," op cit.[32]

BIBLIOGRAPHY: HEALTH AND ILLNESS IN THE NATIVE-AMERICAN (INDIAN) COMMUNITY

Boyd, Doug. *Rolling Thunder*. New York: Random House, 1974.

> An outstanding description of the work of a medicine man and his philosophy is presented.

Brown, Dee. *Bury My Heart at Wounded Knee*. New York: Holt, 1970.

> This book outlines the history of the treaties and battles between the European-American and the Native American.

Deloria, Vine, Jr. *Custer Died for Your Sins: An Indian Manifesto*. New York: Avon Books, 1969.

A description of current philosophies and problems of today's Native Americans is presented by Deloria.

Farnsworth, Dan L. and Rome, Howard P., editors. *Psychiatric Annals* 4 (November 1974).

This special volume of this publication contains several excellent articles regarding the issues and problems of Indian mental health.

Kluckhohn, Clyde. *Navaho Witchcraft.* Boston: Beacon Press, 1944.

Former and current Navaho beliefs regarding witchcraft, its treatment, and its prevention are described.

Kluckhohn, Clyde, and Leighton, Dorothea. *The Navaho.* Garden City, N.Y.: Doubleday, 1962.

This book is a comprehensive anthropologic study of the Navaho. It contains much information regarding health and illness and the prevention and treatment of disease.

Stone, Eric. *Medicine Among the American Indians.* New York: Hafner, 1962.

Multiple treatments for various ailments, as well as a history of these treatments are presented.

FURTHER SUGGESTED READINGS

Books

Bonfante, Leo. *Biographies and Legends of the New England Indians.* Wakefield, Mass.: Pride Publ., 1974.

Cahn, Edgar S., and Hearne, David W., editors. *Our Brother's Keeper: The Indian in White America.* New York: New American Library, 1970.

Deloria, Vine, Jr. *Behind the Trail of Broken Treaties.* New York: Delacourt Press, 1974.

Leighton, Alexander, and Leighton, Dorothea. *The Navaho Door.* Cambridge: Harvard University Press, 1945.

Oaks, Maud; King, Jeff; and Campbell, Joseph. *Where the Two Came to Their Father: A Navaho War Ceremonial.* Princeton, N.J.: Princeton University Press, 1943.

Reichard, Gladys A. *Prayer: The Compulsive Word.* Monograph of The American Ethnological Society. Seattle: University of Washington Press, 1944.

————. *Navaho Religion: A Study of Symbolism.* New York: Pantheon Books, 1950.

Vogel, Virgil. *American Indian Medicine.* Norman, Okla.: University of Oklahoma Press, 1970.

Articles

Allen, James R. "The Indian Adolescent: Psycho-Social Tasks of the Plains Indian of Western Oklahoma." *American Journal of Orthopsychiatry* 43 (April, 1973): 368-375.

Bilagody, Harry. "An American Indian Looks at Health Care." Lecture delivered at the Ninth Training Institute for Psychiatrist-Teachers of Practicing Physicians. Proceedings published by Western Interstate Commission for Higher Education, Boulder, Colo., June, 1969.

Bose, D.P., and Welsh, J.D. "Lactose Malabsorbtion in Oklahoma Indians." *American Journal of Clinical Nutrition* 26 (December 1973): 1320-1322.

Coulehan, John L. "Navaho Indian Medicine: A Dimension in Healing." *Pharos* 39 (July 1976): 93-96.

Cress, J.N., and O'Donnell, J.P. "The Self-esteem Inventory and the Oglala Sioux: A Validation Study." *Journal of Social Psychology* 97 (October 1975): 135-136.

Crowell, Susanne. "Life on the Largest Reservation: Poverty and Progress in the Navajo Nation." *Civil Rights Digest* 6 (Fall 1973): 3-9.

Fortney, Alan Jon. "Has White Man's Lease Expired?" *New England (Boston Sunday Globe)* 23 (January, 1977).

Fuchs, M., and Bashur, R. "Use of Traditional Indian Medicine among Urban Native Americans." *Medical Care* 13 (November 1975): 915-927.

Hardy, Mary Kniep, and Burckhardt, Margaret A. "Nursing the Navaho." *American Journal of Nursing* 77 (January, 1977): 95-96.

Johnson, Carmel-Acosta. "A Case of a Psychotic Navaho Indian Male." In *Social Interaction and Patient Care.* Edited by James K. Skipper, Jr., and Robert C. Leonard. Philadelphia: Lippincott, 1965, pp. 184-195.

Kunitz, S.J. "Navaho and Hopi Fertility 1971-1972." *Human Biology* 46 (September 1974): 435-451.

Maynard, E. "Negative Ethnic Image among Oglala Sioux High School Students." *Pine Ridge Research Bulletin* 6 (December 1968): 18-25.

McCauley, M.A. "Indian Nurse Considers Cultural Traits." *American Journal of Nursing,* May, 1975, pp. 5, 15.

Peretti, Peter O. "Enforced Acculturation and Indian-White Relations." *Indian Historian* 6 (Winter 1973): 38-52.

Primeaux, Martha. "Caring for the American Indian Patient." *American Journal of Nursing* 77 (January 1977): 91-94.

————. "American Indian Health Care Practices: A Cross-Cultural Perspective." *Nursing Clinics of North America* 12 (March 1977): 55-65.

Saland, J.; McNamara, H.; and Cohen, M.I. "Navaho Jaundice: A Variant of Neonatal Hyperbilirubinemia Associated with Breast Feeding." *Journal of Pediatrics* 85 (August 1974): 271-275.

Epilogue

Why must health-care deliverers study ethnicity, culture, and cultural sensitivity? Why must they know the difference between "hot" and "cold" and *yin* and *yang*? Why must they be concerned with the consumer's failure to practice what professionals believe to be good preventive medicine, or with the consumer's failure to comply with a given treatment regimen, or with the consumer's failure to seek medical care during the initial phase of an illness?

There is little disagreement that health-care services in this country are unevenly distributed and that the poor and the ethnic people of color get the short end of the stick in terms of the care they receive (or do not receive). Yet is it often maintained that, when such care *is* provided, these same people fail to utilize it or utilize it inappropriately. Why is this seeming paradox so?

The major focus of this book has been on the provider's and the consumer's differing perceptions of health and illness. These differences may account for the health-care provider's misconception that services are used inappropriately and that people who use them that way do not care about their health. However, what to the casual observer appears to be "misuse" may represent our failure to meet the needs and expectations of the consumer. This possibility may well be difficult for health-care providers to face, but careful analysis of the available information seems to indicate that this may—at least in part—be the case. How, then, can health-care providers change their method of operation and provide both safe and effective care for ethnic people of color and, at the same time, for the population at large? The answer to this question is not an easy one. However, there are a number of measures that can and must be taken to ameliorate the current situation.

1. *Although curricula in professional education are quite full, ethnic studies must be taken by all people who wish to deliver health care.*

It is no longer sufficient to teach a student in the health professions to "accept the patient for who he is." The question arises: Who is he? Introductory sociology and psychology courses fail to provide this information; it is learned best by meeting with the people themselves and letting them describe who they are from their own perspective. I have suggested two approaches to the problem. One is to have ethnic people of color who work as patient advocates or as nurses and physicians come to the class setting and explain how people of their ethnic group view health and illness, and describe the kinds of health care they practice. Another approach is to send students out into communities where they will have the opportunity to meet with people in their own settings. It is not necessary to memorize all the available lists of herbs, hot-cold imbalances, folk diseases, and so forth. The objective is to become more sensitive to the crucial fact that there are multiple factors underlying given patient behaviors. One, of course, is that the patient may well *perceive* and *understand* health and illness from quite a different perspective than that of the health-care provider. Each person comes from a unique culture and a unique socialization process.

2. *The health-care provider must be sensitive to his own perceptions of health and illness, and practices he employs.*

Even though the perceptions of most health professionals are based on a middle-class and medical-model viewpoint, providers must realize that there are other ways of regarding health and illness. The first three chapters of this book are devoted to consciousness-raising about personal self-treatment. It is always an eye-opening experience to publicly scrutinize ourselves in this respect. Quite often we are amazed to see how far we stray from the system's prescribed methods of keeping healthy. The journals confirm that we, too, delay in seeking health care and fail to comply with treatment regimens. Often our ability to comply rests on quite pragmatic issues such as "What is it doing for me?" and "Can I afford to miss work and stay in bed for two days?" As we gain insight into our own health-illness attitudes and behaviors, we tend to be much more sympathetic to and empathetic with the person who fails to come to the clinic or who hates to wait for the physician or who delays in seeking health care.

3. *The health-care provider should be aware of the complex issues that surround the delivery of health care from the patient's viewpoint.*

Calling the medical society for the name of a physician (because a "family member has a health problem") and visiting and comparing the services that are rendered in an urban and a suburban emergency room are exercises that can enable us to better appreciate some of the difficulties that the poor, the ethnic minorities, and the population at large all too often experience when they attempt to obtain health care. Members of the health-care team have a number of advantages in gaining access to the health-care system. For example, they can choose a physician whom they know because they work with him or because someone they work with has recommended him. But health-care providers must never forget that most people do not have these advantages. It is indeed an unsettling, anxiety-provoking, and frustrating experience to be forced to select a physician from a list. It is an even more frustrating experience to be a patient in an unfamiliar location—for example, an urban emergency room, where, quite literally, anything goes.

Another barrier to adequate health care is the financial burden imposed by treatments and tests. However, there are other issues as well. For example, a Chinese patient—who traditionally does not believe that his body replaces blood that is taken for testing purposes—should have as little blood work as necessary, and the reasons for the tests should be carefully explained. A Hispanic woman who believes that taking a pap smear is an intrusive procedure that will bring shame to her should have the procedure performed by a female physician or nurse. When this is not possible, she should have a female chaperone with her for the entire time that the male physician or nurse is in the room.

4. *Every health-care provider must answer the question: Is health a right?*

If health-care providers believe that this is true, then they must be prepared to debate the issue and support reasonable legislation and programs that will bring it to fruition. They must also devote themselves to finding ways of making necessary health care palatable to the consumer. Both the consumer and the health-care team will have to make some adjustments. This cooperative effort will enable the client to become involved in his own treatment.

Another area to be worked through to the satisfaction of both provider and client is the definition of health. Essentially, health-care providers must find a satisfactory definition for *health* or at least accept the fact that the word has several connotations. Perhaps the most salient point is that whatever the individual believes health is, for him that constitutes health. When this concept differs from a standard, middle-class approach, health-care providers must let go of their own bias and accept the unique definition of the client's culture. As suggested earlier, cognizance of one's own *personal* view of health and health care can help atune the professional to other "unconventional" approaches. Furthermore, members of the health-care team must honestly admit that they themselves do not all agree on the definition of "health." Perhaps if this fact is better accepted, health professionals will as a group be able to deal more realistically with health-related problems such as the delivery of care and conflicts about compliance.

5. *More ethnic people of color must be represented in the health-care professions.*

There are multiple issues related to the problem of underrepresentation. Many of the programs designed to increase the number of ethnic people of color in the health-care team have failed. The continued use of the quota system in medical schools is an example of this failure. Difficulties surrounding successful entrance into and completion of professional education programs are complex and numerous, having their roots in impoverished community structures and early educational deprivation. While society is in some ways dealing with such issues—for example, initiating improvements in early education—we are faced with an *immediate* need to bring more ethnic people of color into health-care services.

One method would be the more extensive use of patient advocates and "outreach" workers from the given ethnic community who may be recognized there as healers. These people can provide an overwhelmingly positive service to both the provider and the consumer in that they will serve as the bridge in bringing health-care services to the people. The patient advocate can speak to the client in language that the client understands, and in a manner that is acceptable. Advocates are also able to coordinate medical, nursing, social, and even educational services to meet the patient's needs as he perceives them. In settings where advocates are employed, many problems are resolved to the convenience of both the health-care member and, more importantly, the client!

The nettlesome issue of language bursts forth with regularity. There is always a problem when a non-English-speaking person tries to seek help from the English-speaking majority. The more common languages, French, Italian, and Spanish, should ideally be spoken by at least some of the professional people that staff hospitals, clinics, neighborhood health-care centers, and home health agencies. The use of an interpreter is always difficult because the interpreter generally "interprets" what he translates as he translates. To bring this thought home, the reader should recall the childhood game of "gossip": a message was passed around the room from person to person, and by the time it got back to the sender its content was usually substantially changed. This game is not unlike trying to communicate through an interpreter, and the situation is even more frustrating when—as can often be the case in urban emergency rooms—the interpreter is a 6-year-old child. It is, obviously, far more satisfying and productive if the patient, nurse, and physician can all speak the same language.

6. *Health services must be made far more accessible and available to ethnic people of color.*

I believe that one of the most important events in this modern era of health-care delivery is the advent of neighborhood health centers. They are successful essentially because people who work in them know the people of the neighborhood. In addition, the people of the community can contribute to the decision-making involved in governing and running the agency so that services are tailored to meet the needs of the clients. Concerned members of the health-care team have a moral obligation to support the increased use of health-care centers and *not* their decreased use, as currently tends to occur because of cutbacks in response to allegations (frequently politically motivated) of too-high costs or the misuse of funds. These neighborhood health-care centers provide greatly needed personal services in addition to relief from the widespread depersonalization that occurs in larger institutions. When health-care providers who are genuinely concerned face this reality, perhaps they will be more willing to fight for the survival of these unique centers and strongly urge their increase rather than acquiesce to their demise. In rural areas, the problem is even greater, and far more comprehensive health planning is needed to meet patient needs.

I should like to reiterate that this book was written with the hope that by sharing the material I have been trying to teach, some small changes will be made in the thinking of all health-care providers who read it. There is nothing new in these pages; perhaps it is simply a recombination of material with which the reader is familiar. But I hope it serves its purpose: the sharing of beliefs and attitudes, and the stimulation of lots of consciousness-raising concerning issues of vital concern to health-care providers who must confront the needs of clients with diverse cultural backgrounds.

BIBLIOGRAPHY: EPILOGUE

Branch, Marie Foster, and Paxton, Phyllis Perry. *Providing Safe Nursing Care for Ethnic People of Color.* New York: Appleton, 1976.

> This outstanding book has a threefold purpose: (1) to describe how deficient knowledge about cultural health beliefs impedes health care; (2) to describe a set of approaches to nursing care directed toward the enhancement of *wellness* for ethnic people of color; and (3) to provide models for nursing education.

Brink, Pamela J., editor. *Transcultural Nursing: A Book of Readings.* Englewood Cliffs, N.J.: Prentice-Hall, 1976.

> Transcultural nursing is a blend of anthropology and nursing. The many readings in this book demonstrate this blend in a number of situations.

Epstein, Charlotte. *Effective Interaction in Contemporary Nursing.* Englewood Cliffs, N.J.: Prentice-Hall, 1974.

> Epstein explores what nurses should know about communications; how to deal with stereotypes, such as the "ideal" patient and nurse; the nurse in the community; and the nurse and social change.

Leininger, Madeline. *Nursing and Anthropology: Two Worlds to Blend.* New York: Wiley, 1970.

> In this work we find an overview of transcultural nursing concepts in several settings.

Storlie, Frances. *Nursing and the Social Conscience.* New York: Appleton, 1970.

>   This book helps the reader to look forward and to examine the purpose of nursing and the profession. It offers no answers to the problems of society, but it raises significant questions.

FURTHER SUGGESTED READINGS

Branch, Marie. "Faculty Development to Meet Minority Group Needs: Recruitment, Retention, and Curriculum Change, 1971-1974." Western Interstate Commission for Higher Education, no. 2060.

Group, T.M. "If a Nurse Is to Help in Ghettos." *American Journal of Nursing* 69 (December 1969): 2635-2636.

Hess, Gertrude, and Stroud, Florence. "Racial Tensions: Barriers in Delivery of Nursing Care." *Journal of Nursing Administration* (May-June 1972): 46-49.

La Fargue, Jane. "Role of Prejudice in Rejection of Health Care." *Nursing Research* 21 (January-February 1972): 53-58.

Milio, Nancy. "Values, Social Class, and Community Health Services." *Nursing Research* 16 (Winter 1967): 26-31.

Paxton, Phyllis, and Robinson, Stella P. "Continuing Education Needs of Nurses Serving Minorities and the Poor." *Journal of Continuing Education in Nursing* 5 (March-April 1974): 12-17.

Richeck, H.G. "A Note on Prejudice in Prospective Professional Helpers." *Nursing Research* 19 (March-April 1970): 172-175.

APPENDIX

Suggested Course Outline

NU301. CULTURAL DIVERSITY IN HEALTH AND ILLNESS

The purpose of this course is to bring the student into a direct interface between the ethnic person of color—Black, Chinese, Hispanic, and Native American (Indian)—and the American health-care delivery system. The course content will include discussion of the following topics:

> The perception of health and illness among health-care providers and consumers
> The cultural and institutional factors that affect the consumers' access to and use of health-care resources
> Health-care providers' ways of coping with illness and related problems
> The manner in which ethnic people of color and their problems have been depicted in the literature (e.g.,

From the Boston College School of Nursing, Chestnut Hill, Massachusetts 02167.

the works of Lewis, Kiev, Clark) and their implications for nursing practice.

Goal

The goal of this course is to broaden the student's perception and understanding of health and illness and the variety of meanings it has to the members of ethnic groups of color.

Objectives

Upon completion of this course the student will be able to:

1. Understand more fully the perception and meaning of health and illness to both herself/himself and the ethnic consumer of color.
2. Enter into dialogue with people who have experienced problems in dealing with the American health-care system.
3. Understand the conflicts between the ethnic consumer of color and the American health-care system and its impact on nursing practice and action.
4. Develop ideas as to what nursing practice can do to intervene in this conflict and diminish it.

Texts

The following texts will be read in total and are suggested for purchase:

Branch, Marie Foster, and Paxton, Phyllis Perry. *Providing Safe Nursing Care for Ethnic People of Color.* New York: Appleton, 1976.

Bullough, Bonnie, and Bullough, Vern L. *Poverty, Ethnic Identity, and Health Care.* New York: Appleton, 1972.

Ehrenreich, Barbara, and Ehrenreich, John. *The American Health*

Empire: Power, Profits, and Politics. New York: Vintage Books, 1971.

Assignments and Evaluation

I.	Weekly readings, class attendance, preparedness, and participation	15%
II.	Health interviews	5%
III.	Health diaries	10%
IV.	Reaction papers	20%

The purpose of these papers is to express the student's reactions to the assigned readings up to date of the paper, as well as to the classroom discussion.

| V. | Term paper (maximum 8 to 10 pages) | 25% |

This paper must deal with the problem and issues presented in class and the student's interpretation of how professional nurses must cope with them in practice. All papers must be submitted in proper Turabian format, typed and double spaced.

| VI. | Term project | 25% |

Class presentation, with small group, on perspectives of health and illness in one of the four communities studied; class presentation must include the following data:
1. History of ethnic group in United States.
2. Traditional perceptions of health and illness.
3. Traditional healing methods.
4. Current health-care problems.

Sources must include a bibliography, interviews with people within the given community, and observations.

COURSE OUTLINE

Week I   *Course Introduction: Discussion of General Con-
           cepts of Health*
           Assignments for Class II:
           1. Interview an older member of your family to
              determine (a) what practices were used to pre-
              vent illness and maintain health; (b) what was
              done to treat illness.
           2. Begin a daily diary of your health status for one
              month. (Both assignments must be handed in.)

Week II   *Discussion: Concepts of Illness and Practices for
           Maintaining Health and Preventing Illness*
           Readings:
              *Bullough and Bullough, pp. 1-18
              *Ehrenreich and Ehrenreich, Introduction
              Dubos, *Mirage of Health*
              Dubos, *Man Adapting*

Week III   *The Delivery of Health Care in the United States*
           Readings:
              *Silver, *A Spy in the House of Medicine*
              *Ehrenreich and Ehrenreich, Complete this book
              *Kennedy, *In Critical Condition*

Week IV   *Culture: Its Effect on the Perception of Health and
           Illness*
           Readings:
              *Bullough and Bullough, Complete this book
              *Zola, "Culture and Symptoms: An Analysis of
                 Patients Presenting Complaints"
              *Brink, *Transcultural Nursing*, pp. 93-126

Week V   *Debate and Class Presentation I: Is Health Care a
           Right?*

For complete bibliographic data on the listed readings, see the following Bibliography.
The asterisks indicate required reading.

*Sade, "Medical Care as a Right: A Refutation"

*_____, "National Health Insurance: Rx for Disaster"

*_____, "What About Health Care for the Poor?"

Week VI   *Poverty and Its Impact on Health Care*
Readings:
*Trattner, *From Poor Law to Welfare State*
Freire, *Pedagogy of the Oppressed*
Feagin, *Subordinating the Poor*
Piven, *Regulating the Poor*

Week VII   *Faith and Healing*
Readings:
Kelsey, *Healing and Christianity*
Leek, *Herbs: Medicine and Mysticism*
MacNutt, *Healing*
Film—"We Believe in Nino Fidencio"

Week VIII   *Health and Illness in the Hispanic Communities*
Readings:
*Thomas, *Down These Mean Streets* or *Savior, Savior, Hold My Hand*
*Lewis, *La Vida*
*Lubic, "The Puerto Rican Family"
*Farge, *La Vida Chicana*
Clark, *Health in the Mexican American Culture: A Community Study*
*Branch, Chap. 3

Week IX   *Health and Illness in the Native American Community*
Readings:
Boyd, *Rolling Thunder*
*Deloria, *Custer Died for Your Sins*
Kluckhohn, *The Navaho*
*Branch, Chap. 4
Brown, *Bury My Heart at Wounded Knee*

Week X   *Health and Illness in the Chinese Community*
              Readings:
                  *Li, "Health Care for the Chinese Community in
                      Boston"
                  *Brink, *Transcultural Nursing*, pp. 240-247
                  *Branch, Chap. 5

Week XI   *Health and Illness in the Black Community*
              Readings:
                  Haley, *Roots*
                  *Grier, *Black Rage*
                  Wright, *Black Boy* or *Native Son*
                  *Branch, Chap. 6
                  Gutman, *The Black Family in Slavery and
                      Freedom*
                  Angelou, *I Know Why the Caged Bird Sings*

Week XII   *Institutional Barriers and Advocacy*
              Readings:
                  *Branch, Part I

Week XIII   *Implications for Nursing and Health Care Delivery*
              Readings:
                  *Storlie, *Nursing and the Social Conscience*
                  *Brink, *Transcultural Nursing*, last section, pp.
                      215-275.
                  *Branch, Parts III and IV

Week XIV   *Evaluation and Interethnic Dinner*

Bibliography

Allport, Gordon W. *The Nature of Prejudice* (Abridged). Garden City, New York: Doubleday and Company, Inc., 1958.

Angelou, Maya. *I Know Why The Caged Bird Sings.* New York: Random House, 1970.

Apple, Dorion, ed., *Sociological Studies of Health and Sickness: A Source Book for the Health Professions.* New York: McGraw-Hill, Blakiston Division, 1960.

Arnold, Mark G., and Rosenbaum, Greg. *The Crime of Poverty.* Skokie, Illinois: National Textbook Company, 1973.

Bakan, David. *Disease, Pain and Sacrifice: Toward a Psychology of Suffering.* Chicago: University of Chicago Press, 1968.

Becker, Marshall H. *The Health Belief Model and Personal Health Behavior.* Thorofare, New Jersey, 1974.

Bermann, Eric. *Scapegoat.* Ann Arbor: The University of Michigan Press, 1973.

Branch, Marie Foster and Paxton, Phyllis Perry. *Providing Safe Nursing Care for Ethnic People of Color.* New York: Appleton-Century Crofts, 1976.

Brink, Pamela J., ed. *Transcultural Nursing: A Book of Readings.* Englewood Cliffs, New Jersey: Prentice-Hall, Inc., 1976.

Brown, Dee. *Bury My Heart at Wounded Knee.* New York: Holt, Rinehart and Winston, 1970.

Bullough, Bonnie, and Bullough, Vern L. *Poverty, Ethnic Identity, and Health Care.* New York: Appleton-Century-Crofts, 1972.

Chenault, Lawrence R. *The Puerto Rican Migrant in New York City.* New York: Columbia University Press, 1938.

Clark, Margaret. *Health in the Mexican-American Culture: A Community Study.* Berkeley: University of California Press, 1959.

Crichton, Michael. *Five Patients.* New York: Alfred A. Knopf, 1970.

Davis, Fred, ed. *The Nursing Profession: Five Sociological Essays.* New York: Wiley, 1966.

De Castro, Josue. *The Black Book of Hunger.* Boston: Beacon Press, 1967.

Deloria, Vine Jr. *Custer Died for Your Sins—An Indian Manifesto.* New York: Avon Books, 1969.

Dubos, René Jules, *Man Adapting.* New Haven: Yale University Press, 1965.

———. *Man, Medicine and Environment.* New York: Mentor, 1968.

———. *Mirage of Health.* Garden City, New York: Anchor Book, Doubleday and Company, 1961.

Ehrenreich, Barbara and Ehrenreich, John. *The American Health Empire: Power, Profits, and Politics.* New York: Vintage Books, 1971.

Epstein, Charlotte. *Effective Interaction in Contemporary Nursing.* Englewood Cliffs, New Jersey: Prentice-Hall, Inc., 1974.

Feagin, Joe R. *Subordinating the Poor—Welfare and American Beliefs.* Englewood Cliffs, New Jersey: Prentice-Hall, Inc., 1975.

Finney, Joseph C., ed. *Culture Change, Mental Health and Poverty.* New York: Simon and Schuster, 1969.

Freeman, Howard; Levine, Sol; and Reeder, Leo G., eds. *Handbook of Medical Sociology,* 2nd ed. Englewood Cliffs, New Jersey: Prentice-Hall, Inc., 1972.

Freidson, Eliot. *Profession of Medicine.* New York: Dodd, Mead and Company, 1971.

Freire, Paulo. *Pedagogy of the Oppressed* (trans. Myra Bugman Ramos). New York: The Seabury Press, 1970.

Galdston, Iago. *Medicine and Anthropology.* New York: International Universities Press, Inc., 1959.

Gordon, David M. *Theories of Poverty and Underemployment.* Lexington, Mass.: D. C. Heath and Company, 1972.

Grier, William H., and Cobbs, Price M. *Black Rage.* New York: Bantam Books, 1968.

Gutman, Herbert G. *The Black Family in Slavery and Freedom, 1750-1925.* New York: Pantheon Books, 1976.

Haley, Alex. *Roots.* Garden City, New York: Doubleday and Company, Inc., 1976.

Herzlich, Claudine. *Health and Illness—A Social Psychological Analysis* (trans. Douglas Graham). New York: Academic Press, 1973.

Hickel, Walter J. *Who Owns America?* New York: Paperback Library, 1972 edition.

Illich, Ivan. *Medical Nemesis, The Expropriation of Health.* London: Marion Bogars, 1975.

———— ; Zola, Irving K.; McKnight, John; Caplan, Jonathan; and Shaiken, Harley. *Disabling Professions.* Salem, N.II.. Buyais, 1977.

Jaco, E. Gartly, ed., *Patients, Physicians, and Illness: Sourcebook in Behavioral Science and Medicine.* Glencoe, Illinois: Free Press, 1958.

Jung, Carl G., ed. *Man and His Symbols.* Garden City, New York: Doubleday and Company, Inc., 1964.

Kain, John F., ed. *Race and Poverty, The Economics of Discrimination.* Englewood Cliffs, New Jersey: Prentice-Hall, Inc., 1969.

Kelsey, Morton T. *Healing and Christianity.* New York: Harper and Row, 1973.

Kennedy, Edward M. *In Critical Condition—The Crises in America's Health Care.* New York: Simon and Schuster, 1972.

Kennett, Frances. *Folk Medicine, Fact and Fiction.* New York: Crescent Books, 1976.

Kiev, Ari. *Curanderismo: Mexican-American Folk Psychiatry.* New York: Free Press, 1968.

————. *Magic, Faith, and Healing: Studies in Primitive Psychiatry Today.* New York: Free Press of Glencoe, 1964.

Kluckhohn, Clyde. *Navaho Witchcraft,* Boston: Beacon Press, 1944.

Kluckhohn, Clyde, and Leighton, Dorothea. *The Navaho.* Garden City, New York: Doubleday and Company, Inc., 1962.

Knutson, Andie L. *The Individual, Society and Health Behavior.* New York: Russell Sage Foundation, 1965.

Kosa, John, and Zola, Irving Kenneth. *Poverty and Health — A Sociological Analysis* 2nd ed. Cambridge, Massachusettes: Harvard University Press, 1976.

Kotz, Nick. *Let Them Eat Promises.* Garden City, New York: Doubleday and Company, Inc., 1971.

Leek, Sybil. *Herbs: Medicine and Mysticism.* Chicago: Henry Regnery Company, 1975.

Leff, S., and Leff, Vera. *From Witchcraft to World Health.* New York: The Macmillan Company, 1957.

Leininger, Madeleine. *Nursing and Anthropology: Two Worlds to Blend.* New York: John Wiley and Sons, Inc., 1970.

Lewis, Oscar. *The Children of Sanchez: Autobiography of a Mexican Family.* New York: Random House, 1961.

————. *A Death in the Sanchez Family.* New York: Random House, 1966.

————. *Five Families: Mexican Case Studies in the Culture of Poverty.* New York: The New American Library Basic Books, 1959.

————. *La Vida: A Puerto Rican Family in the Culture of Poverty—San Juan and New York.* New York: Random House, 1966.

Lynch, L. Reddick, ed. *The Cross-Cultural Approach to Health Behavior.* Rutherford, New Jersey: Fairleigh Dickenson University Press, 1969.

MacNutt, Francis. *Healing.* Notre Dame, Indiana: Ave Maria Press, 1974.

————. *The Power to Heal.* Notre Dame, Indiana: Ave Maria Press, 1977.

Mandell, Betty Reid, ed., *Welfare in America: Controlling the "Dangerous Classes."* Englewood Cliffs, New Jersey: Prentice-Hall, Inc. 1975.

Mann, Felix. *Acupuncture—The Ancient Chinese Art of Healing and How It Works Scientifically.* New York: Vintage Books, 1972.

Mechanic, David. *Medical Sociology: A Selective View.* New York: The Free Press, 1968.

Millman, Marcia. *The Unkindest Cut.* New York: William Morrow and Company, Inc., 1977.

Montgomery, Ruth. *Born to Heal.* New York: Coward, McCann, and Geoghegan, 1973.

Newman, Katharine D. *Ethnic American Short Stories.* New York: Pocket Books, 1975.

Norman, John C., ed. *Medicine in the Ghetto.* New York: Appleton-Century-Crofts, 1969.

Opler, Marvin K., ed. *Culture and Mental Health.* New York: The Macmillan Company, 1959.

Osofsky, Gilbert. *Harlem: The Making of a Ghetto.* New York: Harper and Row, 1963.

Padilla, Elena. *Up From Puerto Rico.* New York: Columbia University Press, 1958.

Paul, Benjamin, ed. *Health, Culture, and Community: Case Studies of Public Reactions to Health Programs.* New York: Russell Sage Foundation, 1955.

Pearsall, Marion. *Medical Behavior Science: A Selected Bibliography of Cultural Anthropology, Social Psychology, and Sociology in Medicine.* Louisville: University of Kentucky Press, 1963.

Piven, Frances Fox, and Cloward, Richard A. *Regulating the Poor: The Functions of Public Welfare.* New York: Vintage Books, 1971.

Rand, Christopher. *The Puerto Ricans.* New York: Oxford University Press, 1958.

Read, Margaret. *Culture, Health and Disease.* London: Javistock Publications, 1966.

Roby, Pamela, ed. *The Poverty Establishment.* Englewood Cliffs, New Jersey: Prentice-Hall, Inc., 1974.

Rogler, Lloyd H. *Migrant in the City.* New York: Basic Books, Inc., 1972.

Rude, Donald, ed. *Alienation: Minority Groups.* New York: John Wiley and Sons, Inc., 1972.

Ryan, William. *Blaming the Victim.* New York: Vintage Books, 1971.

Saunders, Lyle. *Cultural Difference and Medical Care: The Case of the Spanish-Speaking People of the Southwest.* New York: Russell Sage Foundation, 1954.

Senior, Clarence. *The Puerto Ricans, Strangers—Then Neighbors.* Chicago: Quadrangle Books, 1961.

Sexton, Patricia Cayo. *Spanish Harlem.* New York: Harper and Row, 1965.

Shih-Chen, Li. *Chinese Medicinal Herbs* (trans. F. Porter Smith and G. A. Stuart). San Francisco: Georgetown Press, 1973.

Shostak, Arthur B.; Van Til, Jon; and Van Til, Sally Bould. *Privilege in America: An End to Inequality?* Englewood Cliffs, New Jersey. Prentice-Hall, Inc., 1973.

Silver, George. *A Spy in the House of Medicine.* Germantown, Maryland: Aspen Systems Corp., 1976.

Simmen, Edward, ed. *Pain and Promise: The Chicano Today.* New York: New American Library, 1972.

Smith, Lillian. *Killers of the Dream.* Garden City, New York: Doubleday and Company, Inc., 1963 edition.

Steiner, Stan. *La Raza—The Mexican Americans.* New York: Harper and Row, 1969.

Stone, Eric. *Medicine Among the American Indians.* New York: Hafner Publishing Company, 1962.

Storlie, Frances. *Nursing and the Social Conscience.* New York: Appleton-Century-Crofts, 1970.

Styron, William. *The Confessions of Nat Turner.* New York: Random House, Inc., 1966.

Tallant, Robert, *Voodoo in New Orleans.* New York: Collier Books, 1974.

Te Selle, Sallie, ed. *The Rediscovery of Ethnicity, Its Implications for Culture and Politics in America.* New York: Harper and Row, 1973.

Thomas, Piri. *Down These Mean Streets.* New York: Signet Books, 1958.

Thomas, Piri. *Savior, Savior, Hold My Hand.* New York: Doubleday and Company, Inc., 1972.

Trattner, Walter I. *From Poor Law to Welfare State: A History of Social Welfare in America.* New York: The Free Press, 1974.

Valentine, Charles A. *Culture and Poverty.* Chicago: The University of Chicago Press, 1968.

Wallnofer, Heinrich, and von Rottauscher, Anna. *Chinese Folk Medicine.* New York: American Library, Inc., 1972.

Wright, Richard. *Black Boy.* New York: Harper and Row, 1937.

_____. *Native Son.* New York: Grosset and Dunlop, 1940.

Zborowski, Mark. *People in Pain.* San Francisco: Jossey-Bass, 1969.

Index